THIRD EDITION

COMPLETELY REVISED & UPDATED

EATING *for* ENDURANCE

ELLEN COLEMAN, RD, MA, MPH

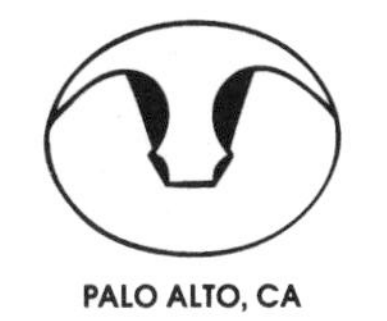

PALO ALTO, CA

Bull Publishing Company
P. O. Box 208
Palo Alto, CA 94302-0208
Phone (415) 322-2855   Fax (415) 327-3300

ISBN 0-923521-13-5

Manufactured in the United States of America.

Distributed to the trade by:
Publishers Group West
4065 Hollis Street
Emeryville, CA 94608

Publisher: James Bull
Production: Myrna Engler/Rogue Valley Publications
Cover Design: Robb Pawlak, Pawlak Design
Cover Photo: Sean Arbabi/Tony Stone Images
Interior Design: Susan Rogin
Composition: Susan Rogin

Library of Congress Cataloging-in-Publication Data

Coleman, Ellen.
Eating for endurance / Ellen Coleman.—3rd ed.
p. cm.
Includes bibliographical references and index.
ISBN 0-923521-13-5 (alk. paper)
1. Athletes—Nutrition. 2. Nutrition. 3. Exercise—Physiological aspects. 4. Energy metabolism. I. Title.
RC 1235.C63 1997
613.2′024796—dc21   96-50205
CIP

Contents

LIST OF FIGURES

LIST OF TABLES

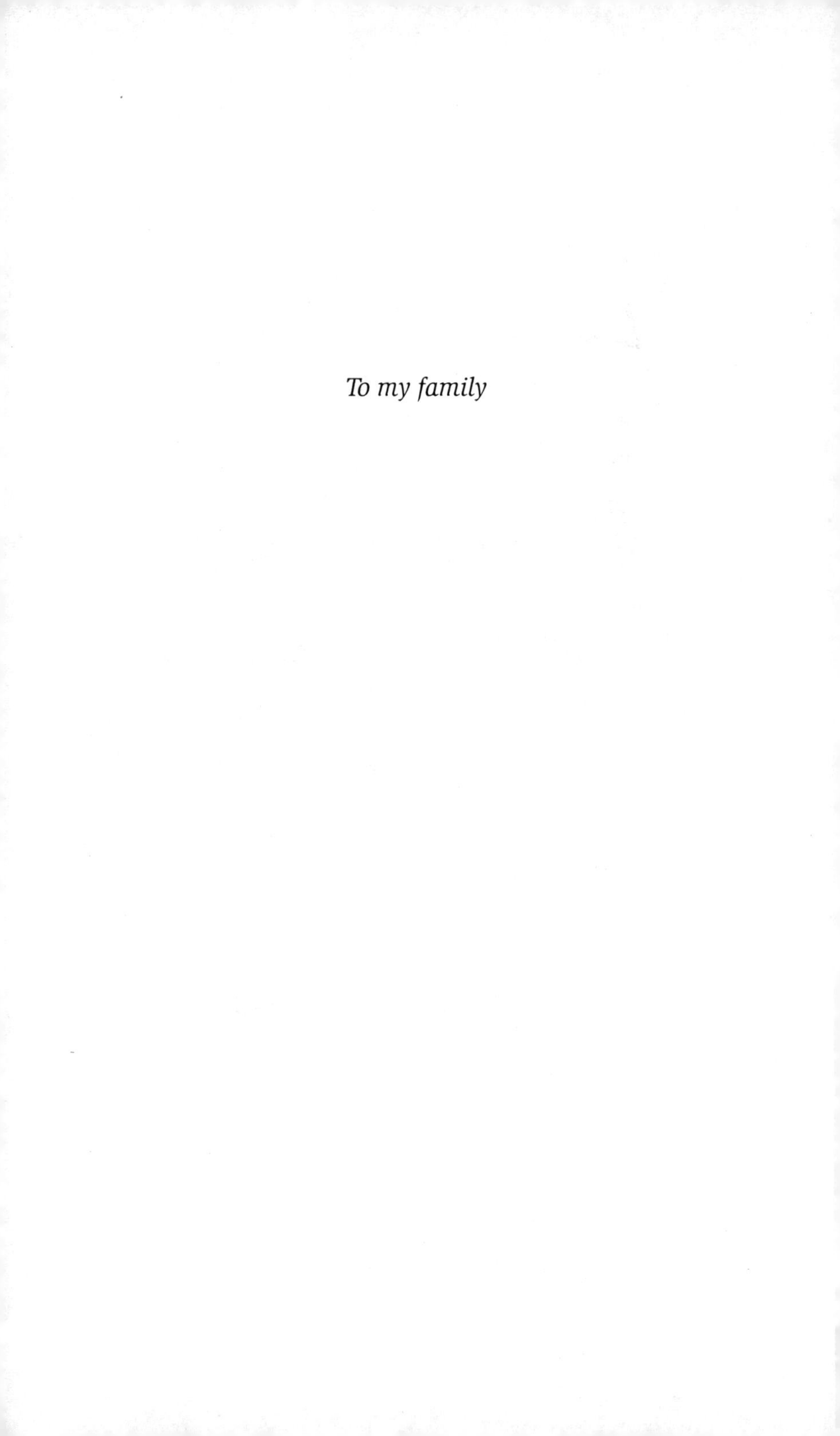

To my family

EATING *for* ENDURANCE

1

Oxygen Is Everything

How Oxygen Use Affects Performance

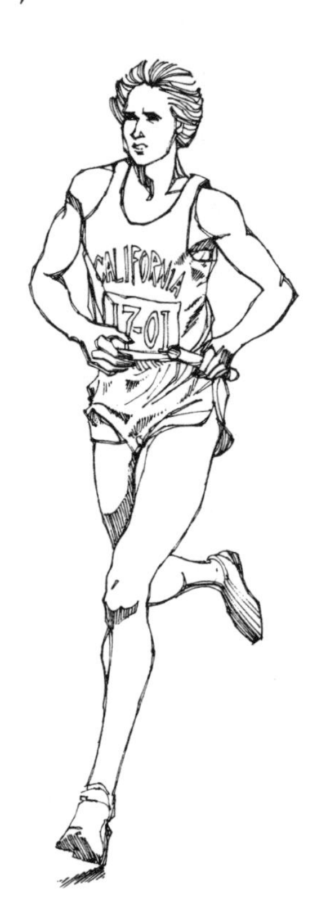

You get out with the front runners, breathing hard. You know you're pushing it, but you feel good. You pass the second mile, still feeling good. You feel proud. You're flying.

At the third mile, you know you're on the way to a record time. You never trained at a pace this fast. It hurts, but you're cruising.

By the fourth mile, though, your running style becomes less fluid. You struggle with the pace. Your legs feel heavy. You have to cut back. When you pass the fifth mile, you're back in control. Your time at the finish is slow, two minutes slower than your average.

This may have been the first time you've gone out front. You stayed ahead of the pack for the first half of the race, and paid for it in the second half. You could have possibly run the same time, or a faster time with less pain if you had paced yourself more evenly.

"But I had a record time at the three-mile mark!" you exclaim. "What happened?"

YOUR BODY'S ABILITY TO USE OXYGEN largely determines your endurance capacity. There are two interrelated energy systems: one dependent on oxygen and the other able to function without oxygen. However, the one that doesn't use oxygen is limited and quickly exhausted. To understand in a general way how these work is important, because it explains how your diet and training influence your performance. This chapter describes the two energy systems and their relationship to the sources of energy in the food we eat.

Metabolism and the Energy Pathways

Our bodies run on food, water, and oxygen. We all know that we need these vital substances, but we don't usually think about how they interact. Many of our ideas (and myths) about sources of energy relate to food. There are plenty of theories in fashion—just ask any health food store clerk. Unfortunately, most of these ideas don't have much to do with how our bodies function.

Although we don't often think about the connection between food and performance, this relationship has a great deal to do with our use of oxygen.

Two related systems supply energy for the body: the *anaerobic* (or lactic-acid) *energy system* that doesn't require oxygen, and the *aerobic energy system* that requires a steady supply of oxygen.

At home or work, your body is probably idling, and you can get by with a minimum amount of food (or calories) and oxygen. When you begin to exercise, however, the demand for energy increases and so does the demand for oxygen. The chemical processes that produce energy take place in the individual cells of your muscles and other tissues.

Chains of chemical reactions utilize oxygen, food, and water to make the body go. This process is referred to as metabolism. Anaerobic metabolism is the series of reactions, requiring no oxygen, that provides immediate energy. It soon needs help, however, from the oxygen-dependent aerobic energy system.

For a brief period of time, about a minute, you can rely on the anaerobic system. In this time, you can exercise at a level that exceeds your ability to make oxygen available to your muscles. Anaerobic metabolism is a built-in survival mechanism—it protects us at moments when we have a sudden need either to fight or flee from danger.

When you exercise longer than several minutes, your body needs a continuous supply of oxygen. Aerobic metabolism provides almost all your energy during exercise that lasts 4 minutes or longer.

The interplay between aerobic and anaerobic energy production is a fascinating part of human performance. Neither the aerobic nor the anaerobic metabolic pathway works exclusively to supply energy during exercise. They work together, each complementing and supporting the other to meet your body's energy demands.

Understanding how the aerobic and anaerobic pathways work together to supply energy will help you determine which fuel the muscles use during a particular exercise. Knowing this will help you appreciate how the food in your diet provides energy for exercise. As a result, you'll be more knowledgeable about choosing foods, training, and pacing yourself for optimal performance.

Food provides you with the fuel for activity. Endurance training increases your body's capacity to utilize oxygen, an action that affects your fuel usage. Pacing also affects how your fuel sources are utilized. So all three—eating, training, and pacing—have an effect on your performance.

ATP—The Energy Currency

An energy-rich compound called adenosine triphosphate (ATP) is used for all energy-requiring processes within your cells. The energy released from the breakdown of ATP is used to power all body functions, such as muscle contraction, so ATP is considered the energy currency of the cell. Another energy-rich compound called creatine phosphate (CP) provides a small reserve of quick energy. The energy released from the breakdown of ATP and CP stores sustains all-out exercise such as sprinting for about 6 to 8 seconds.

To provide a steady supply of energy, ATP must be continually produced. The muscle cells generate and maintain ongoing supplies of ATP, utilizing glucose from carbohydrates, fatty acids from fats, and to a small extent amino acids from proteins. The body extracts the energy from dietary or body stores of carbohydrate, fat, and protein to rebuild the energy-rich ATP.

Carbohydrates and Glucose

Carbohydrates, such as sugar and starch, are the most readily available source of food energy. During digestion and absorption, all carbohydrates are eventually broken down to the simple sugar glucose. Glucose is stored in the muscles and the liver as a substance called glycogen, which is actually a long chain of glucose molecules hooked together. A high-carbohydrate diet is necessary to maintain muscle glycogen—the primary fuel for most sports.

Although the carbohydrate in food eaten before and during exercise can supply energy by increasing your blood sugar, your main energy source is the muscle glycogen you have stored ahead of time. After 90 to 120 minutes, your performance may begin to deteriorate as your muscle glycogen stores are depleted. Training and diet affect how much muscle glycogen you can store. Training and pacing determine how rapidly it is used up during exercise.

There is a two-stage chemical process to break down glucose for energy, shown in Figure 1-1 on page 9.

The Anaerobic Pathway

Glucose is the only fuel that can be used when oxygen is not available. In the anaerobic pathway, glucose is broken down to a substance called pyruvate. In the absence of oxygen, this pyruvate is converted to lactic acid, forming 2 molecules of ATP. When oxygen is available, pyruvate is broken down for energy in the aerobic pathway.

Although the anaerobic pathway provides energy quickly, there is a limit to the amount of lactic acid the body can tolerate. High levels make the muscle more acidic, and this acid interferes with muscle contraction and energy production. For this reason, anaerobic metabolism can fuel exercise for only a short period of time (about a minute). When oxygen becomes available, lactic acid is converted back into pyruvate or burned directly by the muscles for energy. Lactic acid can also go to the liver and be converted back into glucose.

The anaerobic pathway provides us with the energy for all-out efforts lasting up to 60 seconds, such as long sprints. It also provides energy for the bursts that are common in sports like soccer, basketball, football, and tennis.

The Aerobic Pathway

Aerobic metabolism depends on a continuous supply of oxygen. When oxygen is available, glucose can be broken down far more efficiently, without being converted to lactic acid. When glucose is broken down in the aerobic pathway, 36 ATP molecules are produced. This is 18 times more energy than when glucose is converted to lactic acid in the anaerobic pathway.

Amino acids (from proteins) and fatty acids (from fat) can also go through the aerobic pathway to provide energy. However, protein and fat cannot provide energy without the presence of oxygen. This means that when oxygen is limited, glucose (from carbohydrate) is the only fuel available for energy production.

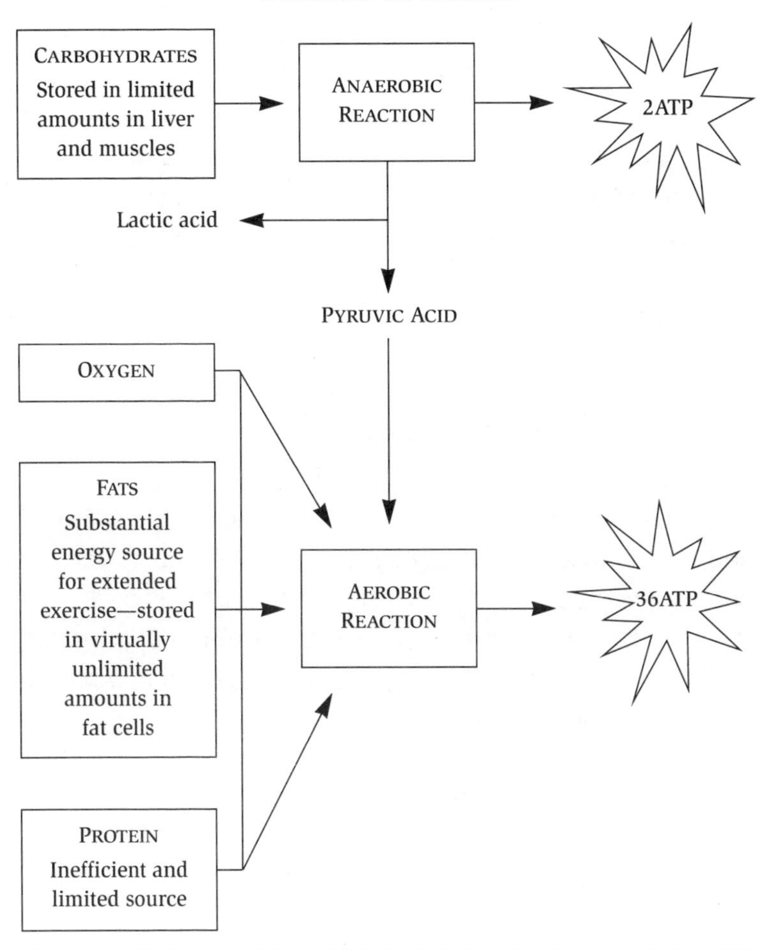

FIGURE 1-1. The anaerobic and aerobic systems work together to provide energy for the body. When enough oxygen is present in the muscle, the more efficient aerobic reaction system operates to provide the energy (ATP) used for muscle contraction. This system can also utilize fats and, to a lesser extent, proteins that are stored in virtually unlimited amounts in the body. The aerobic system is very efficient and can produce up to 18 times the amount of ATP produced by the anaerobic system. The anaerobic system contributes most during exercise periods of only 1 or 2 minutes.

Amino acids are not a primary energy source during exercise. Their regular functions are for body tissue growth and repair (see Chapter 7). However, the body will use protein for energy if a person is not eating enough calories or carbohydrates (i.e., the individual is on a starvation diet or is fasting).

Fatty acids, like amino acids, cannot support high-intensity exercise. However, fat is a very important energy source for prolonged endurance exercise (see Chapters 3 and 6). And unlike carbohydrate, fat is stored in vast quantities.

The Aerobic/Anaerobic Combination

At the beginning of exercise, time is needed for the heart and blood vessels to get oxygen-rich blood to the muscles and for the muscles to extract oxygen from the blood. (Thus the importance of a proper pre-event warm-up.) During this lag time (about a minute), anaerobic ATP production provides most of the energy for the exercise.

After several minutes, aerobic ATP production provides most of the energy needed to sustain exercise. However, when the exercise becomes too intense for enough energy to be produced aerobically (as when you are running up a hill or sprinting in a marathon), the anaerobic pathway will be pulled in to meet the deficit. This additional ATP is bought at the price of increasing the level of lactic acid, which causes a more rapid breakdown of muscle glycogen.

In an event lasting 2 minutes, the contributions of aerobic and anaerobic metabolism are about equal. As the distance (or time) increases, the contribution of aerobically produced energy increases (see Figure 1-2 on page 12).

Although anaerobic energy production determines performance during sprint-type activities, the capacity to produce ATP aerobically determines someone's endurance performance. Thus, the availability of oxygen in large part determines a person's potential for aerobic exercise.

Your capacity for exercise intensity and for duration are inversely related. As the distance increases, you have to reduce your intensity, or pace. For example, a runner can't run a marathon (26.2 miles) as fast as a 10-kilometer (K) race (6.2 miles). You can only perform at a certain percentage of your maximum aerobic capacity for any given distance or time.

The aerobic pathway simply cannot tolerate the same level of intensity as the distance increases. For example, a trained distance runner can run a mile at 100% of his aerobic capacity. In a 5K run, he can use about 95% of his aerobic capacity. In a 10K run, he can average about 90% of his aerobic capacity. In the marathon, he can use only 60% to 80% of his aerobic capacity.

There is an additional reason that you cannot perform close to your aerobic capacity during prolonged endurance events. When endurance exercise exceeds 90 to 120 minutes, your muscle glycogen stores become progressively lower. When they drop to critically low levels, you feel exhausted and must either stop exercising or continue at a much slower pace. Muscle glycogen depletion is a well-recognized limitation to endurance performance and is discussed further in Chapters 4 and 5.

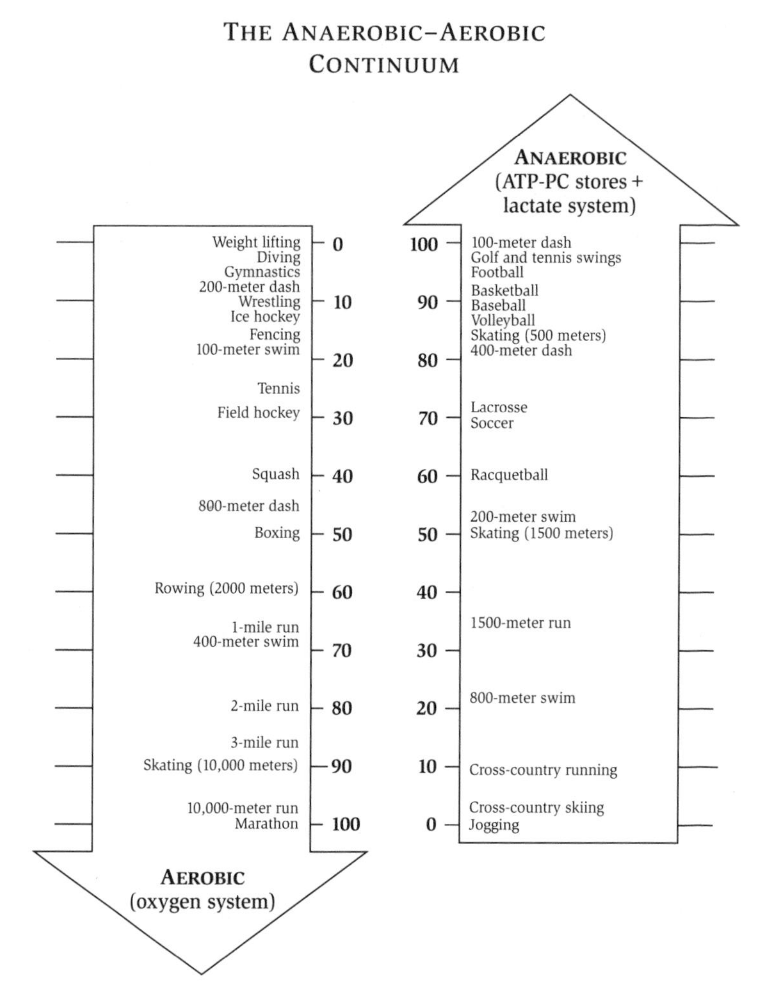

FIGURE 1-2. Whereas the 100-meter dash is considered a pure anaerobic event and the marathon a pure aerobic event, most other activities use ATP from both systems. Athletes should train both systems in accordance with the demands of their sport.

Pacing

How can you influence your body to utilize your fuel sources more efficiently? One way is to control the intensity or pace of the exercise so that sufficient oxygen will be continuously available to the muscles.

Even in shorter events such as a 10K race, pace is extremely important. If you go out too fast, too much lactic acid will accumulate in your blood and the advantage you gained with the early speed will be more than offset by your sub-par performance in the rest of the race. This is what happened to the runner in the story at the beginning of the chapter.

In longer events such as the marathon, going out too fast will result in more rapid glycogen depletion and you'll hit the wall sooner. As you'll see in Chapters 3 and 6, proper pacing increases the use of fat as fuel so that muscle glycogen is spared. Slowing down muscle glycogen utilization enhances your endurance.

Ultimately, the aerobic and anaerobic pathways will determine whether you finish your event, how well you finish, and the intensity at which you perform throughout the event. As you'll see, what you eat and drink before and during the event will also affect your ability to get the most out of your energy sources.

2

The Golden Standard of Physical Fitness

Measuring Your Capacity to Use Oxygen

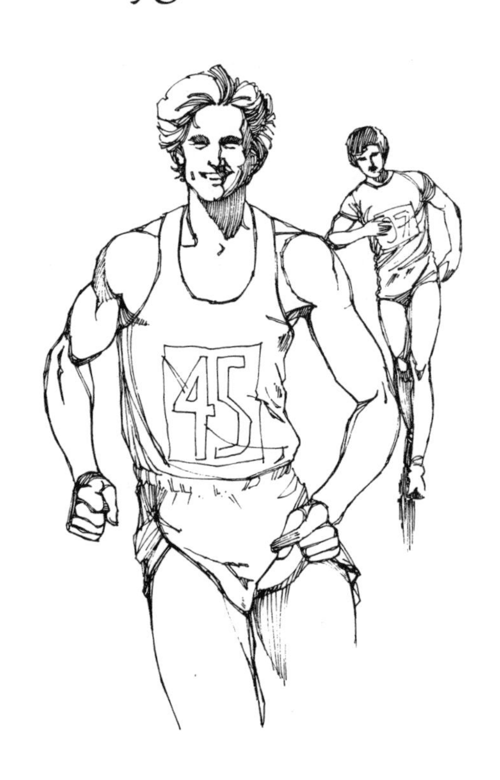

You and your running buddy have almost identical times in the mile and trade off leads in the 10K.

You both decide to run a marathon, and you train together for it by putting in many long, comfortable runs. After tapering off on your mileage, you both load up on carbohydrates for the event.

On the day of the marathon, you run together for the first 10 miles. Your buddy has a tough time keeping the pace after that, but you feel good. Finally, he tells you to take off, and you leave your friend behind.

You finish the race with no problems and wait at the finish line. Finally, he walks in and you ask, "What happened?"

"When I hit the twenty-first mile, I felt terrible," he said. "I could only walk."

Later, over dinner, you rehash the race. "How come," he laments, "I can run with you in a 10K but not in a marathon?"

YOU KNOW THE IMPORTANCE of oxygen for endurance exercise. You also know that lactic acid build-up can limit your ability to perform. Because both these factors are so important, we'll discuss how your capacity to use oxygen and the level at which your muscles accumulate lactic acid can both be used to predict your performance capacity.

Maximal Oxygen Consumption

The harder you exercise, the more oxygen you require. The amount of oxygen that your body uses is directly related to the intensity of the exercise.

However, there is a point beyond which your use of oxygen will not increase, even when the intensity of the exercise continues to increase. The value at which your oxygen consumption plateaus is called your maximal oxygen consumption (abbreviated $\dot{V}O_{2max}$); $\dot{V}O_{2max}$ is a scientific measurement of your aerobic capacity and is regarded as the best criterion of endurance capacity and physical fitness. A person with a high $\dot{V}O_{2max}$ can exercise harder and longer than a person with a low $\dot{V}O_{2max}$.

The delivery of oxygen by the cardiovascular system and the extraction of oxygen from the blood by the muscles determine the $\dot{V}O_{2max}$.

A large person will use more total oxygen because he*

*To avoid the awkwardness of using him or her, the masculine form is used unless the context calls for the feminine.

has more oxygen-requiring tissue. To accommodate individual differences in size, $\dot{V}O_{2max}$ values are calculated to account for differences in body weight. A person's maximal oxygen usage (measured in liters per minute) is divided by his weight measured in kilograms (1 kilogram is equal to 2.2 pounds). $\dot{V}O_{2max}$ values are expressed in milliliters of oxygen used per kilogram of body weight per minute (abbreviated ml/kg/min).

Values for sedentary college-age males and females are in the mid 40 and 30 ml/kg/min, respectively. Male endurance athletes (runners, cyclists, triathletes, swimmers) generally have $\dot{V}O_{2max}$ values in the 60s, and elite male endurance athletes have values in the 70 to 80 ml/kg/min. Female endurance athletes are usually in the 50s and elite female endurance athletes are in the 60 to 70 ml/kg/min.

Your ultimate aerobic capacity seems to be genetically determined, but whether you reach your full potential will depend on training. An untrained person can improve his $\dot{V}O_{2max}$ by 15% or 20% with endurance training.

We define endurance exercise as exercising for at least 3 days per week, for 30 minutes, at 75% of $\dot{V}O_{2max}$ (about 80% of maximum heart rate). Aerobic capacity peaks within 6 months to 2 years following the initiation of an endurance exercise program. However, even after your $\dot{V}O_{2max}$ has stopped increasing, you can continue to improve your performance. Why?

$\dot{V}O_{2max}$ and Performance

Elite athletes can exercise at their $\dot{V}O_{2max}$ for only about 8 to 10 minutes. This means that most of the time we are exercising at a percentage of our aerobic capacity (e.g., 95% in a 5K run, 60% to 80% in a marathon). Even when your $\dot{V}O_{2max}$ no longer increases, you can continue to improve by developing your ability to tax a higher percentage of your aerobic capacity.

In practical terms, you can complete the same distance at a faster speed for the same effort. Whereas most marathon runners run at a pace that requires 60% to 80% of their $\dot{V}O_{2max}$, elite marathoners can run the distance at over 85% of their $\dot{V}O_{2max}$.

An example of one such athlete is Alberto Salazar, a former world record holder in the marathon. His $\dot{V}O_{2max}$ was 70 ml/kg/min, below that expected based on his world record performance of 2 hours and 8 minutes. However, Salazar was able to run a marathon at 86% of his $\dot{V}O_{2max}$, a percentage much higher than that of other runners.

These figures demonstrate that an athlete with a $\dot{V}O_{2max}$ below that of his competitors may be able to outperform them by being able to work closer to his $\dot{V}O_{2max}$. However, training does have its limits—the genetically well-endowed athlete who can work close to his $\dot{V}O_{2max}$ will continue to have the edge over the less well-endowed athlete.

Women—nonathletes and athletes alike—have lower aerobic capacities than men. Women carry a greater percentage of their body weight as fat compared to men. This sex-specific essential body fat is the major reason that women have lower $\dot{V}O_{2max}$ values. Women also have less total hemoglobin and so the oxygen content of the blood delivered to their muscles is lower.

When $\dot{V}O_{2max}$ is expressed relative to the fat-free mass or active muscle mass (rather than body weight), the differences between the sexes almost disappear. However, women must still move their entire body weight (muscle and fat), so their performance is affected accordingly. However, highly trained female endurance athletes have $\dot{V}O_{2max}$ values only about 10% lower than those of highly conditioned male endurance athletes.

The Lactate Threshold

The lactate threshold may explain why endurance training results in the ability to tax a higher percentage of your $\dot{V}O_{2max}$ It may also explain why some athletes can use a higher percentage of $\dot{V}O_{2max}$ than others during endurance exercise.

The lactate threshold is the point during exercise of increasing intensity at which lactic acid begins to accumulate in your blood. It is usually expressed as a percentage of $\dot{V}O_{2max}$.

Untrained people have lactate thresholds (they begin to accumulate lactic acid in the blood) at about 50% of their $\dot{V}O_{2max}$. Trained people have lactate thresholds at about 70% of their $\dot{V}O_{2max}$. This higher level for lactic acid accumulation means that trained people can exercise at a higher percentage of their $\dot{V}O_{2max}$.

An athlete with a lactate threshold at 80% of his $\dot{V}O_{2max}$ should have a better endurance potential than an athlete with the same $\dot{V}O_{2max}$ but a lactate threshold at 70%. The higher percentage indicates that he can work closer to his aerobic capacity without accumulating lactic acid.

An athlete's lactate threshold is a better predictor of endurance performance lasting 30 minutes to 4 hours than is the athlete's $\dot{V}O_{2max}$. This is because the athlete's lactate threshold is a better indicator of the athlete's ability to sustain a high rate of energy expenditure during prolonged exercise. In fact, the running speed at which the athlete's lactate threshold occurs is a much better predictor of marathon performance than is the athlete's $\dot{V}O_{2max}$.

Remember the two marathon runners in the story at the beginning of the chapter? Although their $\dot{V}O_{2max}$ values were the same, and they could run a 10K race together, the athlete with the higher lactate threshold performed better in the marathon. He accumulated less lactic acid and had a slower rate of muscle glycogen depletion, qualities that enabled him to maintain a faster running speed throughout the entire race.

In contrast, a 10K race does not last long enough to be limited by muscle glycogen depletion. We discuss this further in Chapter 3.

As with $\dot{V}O_{2max}$, genetics and training both appear to influence the lactate threshold. The type of endurance training that increases $\dot{V}O_{2max}$ also increases the blood lactate threshold.

Your $\dot{V}O_{2max}$ and lactate threshold can be measured during a graded exercise test on a bicycle or treadmill. Although $\dot{V}O_{2max}$ can be estimated from graded exercise tests or field tests (e.g., a 1 1/2-mile run), the lactate threshold must be measured. Many sports medicine facilities, colleges, and hospitals offer such tests.

3

What Determines Fuel Usage?

Your Body's Use of Glycogen and Fat

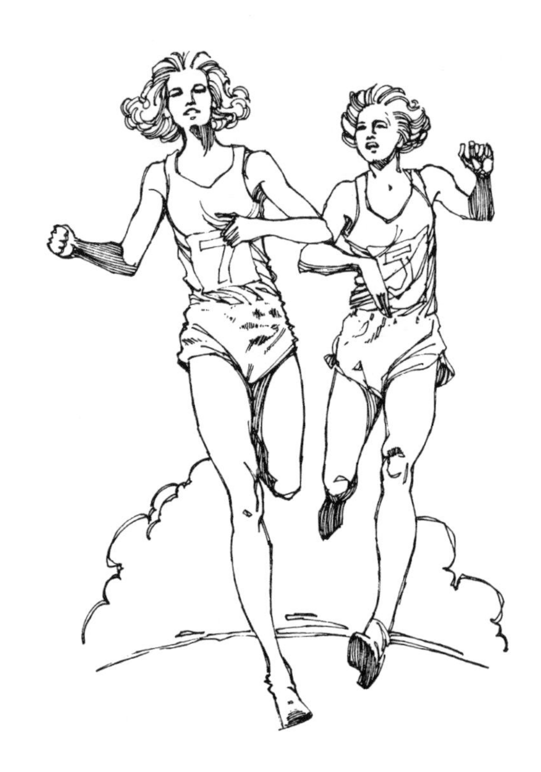

two of my friends were competing in the same marathon. I expected them to finish in about the same time—based on their performances in other races and their comparable times during marathon training. One went out faster than she had planned and passed the half-marathon mark 5 minutes ahead of schedule. The other woman came through the half-marathon point right on her predicted pace. By 20 miles, the woman who had gone out slower passed the woman who had thought she was "putting money in the bank" by going out so fast.

The woman who paced herself finished comfortably and was several minutes ahead of her predicted time. The woman who went out too fast finished in agony, several minutes slower than her target time.

YOUR GOAL IS TO SUPPLY ENERGY to the muscle and you have two major fuels—glycogen (your high-octane fuel) and fat. A variety of factors determine which type of fuel your muscles will use during exercise. These include the intensity of the exercise, the duration of the exercise, your training level, and the composition of your diet.

Intensity

The intensity of the exercise is particularly important in determining the energy source your muscles will use. Exercise that is intense in nature and lasts a fairly short time (such as sprinting) depends principally on the anaerobic pathway for energy. For such exercise, only glucose, derived principally from the breakdown of muscle glycogen, can be used for fuel.

As noted in Chapter 1, glucose used aerobically (during exercise of low to moderate intensity) will provide 18 times the energy of glucose used anaerobically. Thus, with use of the anaerobic energy system, muscle glycogen is being used 18 times faster than when glucose is used aerobically. This rapid rate of glycogen breakdown will also occur during high-intensity exercise (i.e., over 70% $\dot{V}O_{2max}$) when the anaerobic pathway is pulled in to assist the aerobic pathway to provide adequate ATP. (An example would be a sprint during a marathon.)

Extended mixed anaerobic-aerobic intermittent exercise like soccer, basketball, football drills, and running and swimming intervals also causes a greater breakdown of muscle glycogen.

What about aerobic exercise such as distance running? Muscle glycogen and blood glucose supply half the energy for a moderate workout (at or below 60% of $\dot{V}O_{2max}$) and supply nearly all the energy for a hard workout (above 80% of $\dot{V}O_{2max}$).

Exercise of low to moderate intensity (up to 60% of $\dot{V}O_{2max}$) can be fueled almost entirely aerobically. The hormonal changes that occur with exercise—increased epinephrine (adrenaline) and decreased insulin levels—cause your fat (adipose) tissue to release fatty acids into the bloodstream. These fatty acids, combined with fat pools within the muscle, supply about half the energy demands for low- to moderate-intensity exercise. Glycogen and blood glucose supply the rest.

There are several reasons that fat cannot be used as fuel during high-intensity exercise (above 70% of $\dot{V}O_{2max}$). First, the breakdown of fat to ATP is a slow process and cannot supply ATP rapidly enough to provide energy for high-intensity exercise.

Also, glucose provides more calories per liter of oxygen than does fat. Glucose delivers 5.10 calories per liter of oxygen and fat delivers 4.62 calories per liter of oxygen. When less oxygen becomes available, as during high-intensity exercise, using glucose gives the muscles a distinct advantage because less oxygen is needed to produce energy.

The shift in fuel from glycogen to fat as the exercise intensity increases is partly due to the accumulation of lactic acid. During high-intensity exercise, lactic acid hinders the muscles in their attempt to use fat. Thus, the muscles must rely more on glycogen for energy production.

A word on pacing: Because intense exercise requires muscle glycogen as fuel, whereas moderate exercise can be fueled by essentially limitless fatty acids, any sparing of muscle glycogen will result in increased endurance. This is the physiological basis for choosing a pace that can be maintained for long periods of time.

Remember the two women marathon runners at the beginning of the chapter? The one who set the fast initial pace succumbed to glycogen depletion earlier than usual. The woman who paced herself was able to delay glycogen depletion and run a personal best.

You use more glycogen than necessary by going out too fast in a race and by continuing at a pace that is too fast. To put it another way, your optimal long-term pace will be at the speed that allows you to burn more fat and less carbohydrate. (See Table 3-1 for the relationship between distance and energy sources.)

TABLE 3-1
RELATIONSHIP BETWEEN DISTANCE AND ENERGY SOURCES

DISTANCE OF RACE	O_2 CONSUMPTION (% OF $\dot{V}O_{2MAX}$)	GLYCOGEN CONTRIBUTION	FAT
Marathon	75%	70%	30%
30 Kilometers	78%	70%	30%
20 Kilometers	80%	70%	30%
15 Kilometers	81%	75%	25%
10 Kilometers	83%	80%	20%
5 Kilometers	90%	95%	5%
800 Meters	100%	100%	0%

Duration

The duration of exercise also determines whether the fuel used will be muscle glycogen or fat. The longer your exercise, the greater will be the contribution of fat as fuel. Fat can supply as much as 60% to 70% of the energy needed during moderate-intensity exercise lasting from 4 to 6 hours.

As the duration of the exercise increases, the intensity must decrease, as there is a limited supply of stored glycogen. When muscle glycogen stores are low, fat breakdown supplies most of the energy needed for exercise. However, fat can be used for fuel only to about 60% of $\dot{V}O_{2max}$. Also, a certain level of carbohydrate breakdown is necessary for fat to be burned for energy. To this extent, fat burns in a carbohydrate flame.

As a result of the relationship between exercise intensity and duration, muscle glycogen is the predominant fuel for most types of exercise. It takes at least 20 minutes of continuous exercise for fat to be available as fuel in the form of free fatty acids. Most people don't train long enough to burn significant amounts of fat during the exercise itself. Also, most people train and compete at 70% of $\dot{V}O_{2max}$ or above, which limits the use of fat as fuel.

This does not mean that a person needs to work out for a long time at a low intensity to lose body fat. When the workout creates a caloric deficit, the body will pull from its fat stores at a later time to make up that caloric deficit. The role of exercise for body fat loss is discussed in Chapter 14.

Training Level

Your $\dot{V}O_{2max}$ will also determine what fuel your muscles use during exercise. Remember—the delivery of blood by the heart and extraction of oxygen from the muscles determine your $\dot{V}O_{2max}$. Endurance training increases both the maximum delivery of blood by the heart and the extraction of oxygen from the blood by the muscles.

Thus, endurance training increases your ability to perform more aerobically at the same absolute level of exercise (e.g., running 8 miles per hour). This means that you can use more fat and less glycogen at the same absolute level of exercise.

Untrained people have a lactate threshold (they start to accumulate lactic acid in the blood) at about 50% of their $\dot{V}O_{2max}$. Trained people have a lactate threshold at about 70% of their $\dot{V}O_{2max}$. Lactic acid speeds up the rate of muscle glycogen depletion by interfering with the muscle's use of fat as fuel. Having a higher lactate threshold is another reason that trained people use more fat and less glycogen at the same absolute level of exercise.

Endurance training also increases the ability of the aerobic energy system in your muscles to use fat for energy. When more fat is burned, less glycogen is used. This glycogen sparing effect of fat utilization is beneficial during prolonged exercise because muscle glycogen depletion limits endurance.

Last, endurance training increases the capacity of your muscles to store glycogen. Thus, endurance training confers a double performance advantage: Your muscle glycogen stores are higher at the onset of exercise, and you deplete them at a slower rate.

Compare two athletes; one has a $\dot{V}O_{2max}$ of 70 milligrams per kilogram per minute (ml/kg/min) and the other has a $\dot{V}O_{2max}$ of 65 ml/kg/min. They both have lactate thresholds at 75% of their $\dot{V}O_{2max}$ values—meaning that the athlete with the higher $\dot{V}O_{2max}$ also has the higher lactate threshold. The athlete with the higher $\dot{V}O_{2max}$ and lactate threshold will use less glycogen at the same running speed than the athlete with the lower $\dot{V}O_{2max}$. The athlete with the higher $\dot{V}O_{2max}$ will deplete his glycogen stores more slowly.

On the other hand, if the athlete with the lower $\dot{V}O_{2max}$ trained himself to the point that his anaerobic threshold came at a higher percentage of his $\dot{V}O_{2max}$, he could make up the difference in performance. If his anaerobic threshold occurred at the same absolute workload (e.g., at 8 miles per hour) as that of the athlete with the higher $\dot{V}O_{2max}$, the two athletes would tend to have the same endurance potential.

Diet

The percentages of carbohydrate and fat in your diet also determine the amount of glycogen and fat used as fuel. If your diet is high in carbohydrate, you'll use more glycogen as fuel. If your diet is high in fat, you'll use more fat as fuel.

This does not mean that you should eat a high-fat diet. Even the leanest athletes have more fat stored than they'll ever need during exercise. The goal is to increase your utilization of fat. You can do this far more effectively and healthfully by endurance training than by eating a high-fat diet. This is discussed further in Chapter 6.

Keep in mind that eating too much fat decreases your

carbohydrate intake. As the next chapter indicates, eating a low-carbohydrate diet decreases your muscle glycogen stores. Lower muscle glycogen reserves decrease your ability to sustain high-intensity exercise and limit your endurance.

Maximum glycogen storage depends on a combination of diet and training (endurance training permits greater glycogen storage). Thus, the ideal diet supplies enough carbohydrate (6 to 10 grams of carbohydrate per kilogram of body weight daily—about 60% to 70% of calories) to ensure optimal muscle glycogen stores. We discuss this further in the next chapter.

4

Recommended Training Diet

Eating for Both Health and Performance

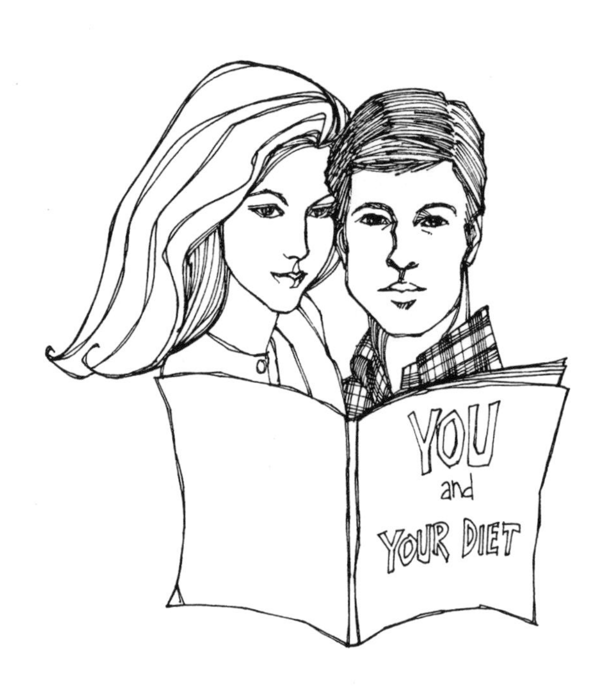

A friend of mine was training for a 200-mile bicycle ride. A week before the event, he headed out for a hilly, 100-mile workout. He noticed that his legs felt stiff and heavy but thought he'd loosen up on the ride. He struggled to complete the first climb, standing up in his lowest gear on a grade he could normally surmount with ease. At the top of the hill, he gave up and headed home.

When we met over dinner that evening, he was about to give up on his 200-mile attempt. I told him to rest a day and eat a high-carbohydrate diet while tapering his training for the remainder of the week. He finished the 200-mile ride in his best time ever.

My friend had succumbed to training glycogen depletion.

REPLENISHING AND MAINTAINING muscle glycogen stores during intensive training require a carbohydrate-rich diet. Adequate muscle glycogen stores allow you to exercise harder and longer with less fatigue. A high-carbohydrate, low-fat diet is also recommended to promote optimum health. The dietary guidelines developed to promote health establish a good foundation for athletes who desire peak performance.

Glycogen Stores and Training

Have you ever had days of training when you felt that you'd lost endurance, speed, and precision? Many such bad days are caused by low levels of glycogen in your muscles.

Most people think that muscle glycogen depletion occurs only during prolonged endurance exercise like marathon running. Glycogen depletion can also be a gradual process, occurring over repeated days of heavy training when muscle glycogen breakdown exceeds its replacement. When this happens, your glycogen stores drop lower with each successive day, and your workouts become more difficult and less enjoyable.

It's normal to be tired after several days of high-intensity workouts, especially if you train several hours a day. However, muscle glycogen depletion (and/or dehydration) should be suspected when you're always tired and unable to maintain your usual training intensity. The deterioration in performance and feeling of sluggishness associated with glycogen depletion is often referred to as "staleness."

A sudden weight loss of several pounds (due to glycogen and water loss) often accompanies training glycogen depletion. When you don't consume enough carbohydrate or calories and/or don't take days off to rest, you're a prime candidate.

Carbohydrate Recommendations for Training

Training glycogen depletion can be prevented by a carbohydrate-rich diet (6 to 10 grams of carbohydrate per kilogram of body weight) and periodic rest days to give the muscles time to rebuild their stores. The typical American diet (46% carbohydrate or about 4 to 5 grams of carbohydrate per kilogram of body weight) doesn't supply enough carbohydrate. Carbohydrate is essential for glycogen synthesis and should provide at least 6 grams of carbohydrate per kilogram of body weight daily (about 60% of your total calories).

A diet containing 8 to 10 grams of carbohydrate per kilogram of body weight per day (about 65% to 70% carbohydrate) is recommended when you're training hard (70% of $\dot{V}O_{2max}$ or more) for several hours or more. However, if you're exercising for an hour or less, a diet containing 6 grams of carbohydrate per kilogram of body weight per day is sufficient to replenish your glycogen stores. By keeping your carbohydrate intake high, you can minimize the chronic fatigue that results from muscle glycogen depletion.

A diet providing 8 to 10 grams of carbohydrate per kilogram of body weight per day may require that you reduce your fat intake to 20% to 25% of total calories. When your carbohydrate requirements are high, you can increase your sugar intake, but about half of your calories should continue to come from complex carbohydrates.

The recommendations for carbohydrate are given in grams per kilogram because this is an easy way to determine how much you need. For example, a 154-pound person (70 kg) who trains strenuously for an hour needs 420 grams of carbohydrate daily. You can determine the carbohydrate content of different foods by reading food labels.

A Healthy Diet Emphasizes Carbohydrates

In addition to providing adequate muscle glycogen stores, a healthy diet should help to prevent heart disease, stroke, and cancer. You can meet both objectives by following the Food Guide Pyramid and the 1995 Dietary Guidelines for Americans. The Dietary Guidelines for Americans (developed by a joint committee of the U.S. Department of Agriculture and the U.S. Department of Health and Human Services) are designed to reduce the risk of chronic disease. The Food Guide Pyramid is based on these recommendations. The guidelines are listed below.

The Seven Dietary Guidelines

Eat a variety of foods.

Balance the food you eat with physical activity. Maintain or improve your weight.

Choose a diet with plenty of grain products, vegetables, and fruit.

Choose a diet low in fat, saturated fat, and cholesterol.

Choose a diet moderate in sugars.

Choose a diet moderate in salt and sodium.

If you drink alcoholic beverages, do so in moderation.

The Food Guide Pyramid (Figure 4-1) shows the foods that should be included in a healthful diet and in what amounts. The grain group forms the base of the pyramid, the fruit and vegetable groups are on the second tier, and the meat and dairy groups are on the third tier. Because fats

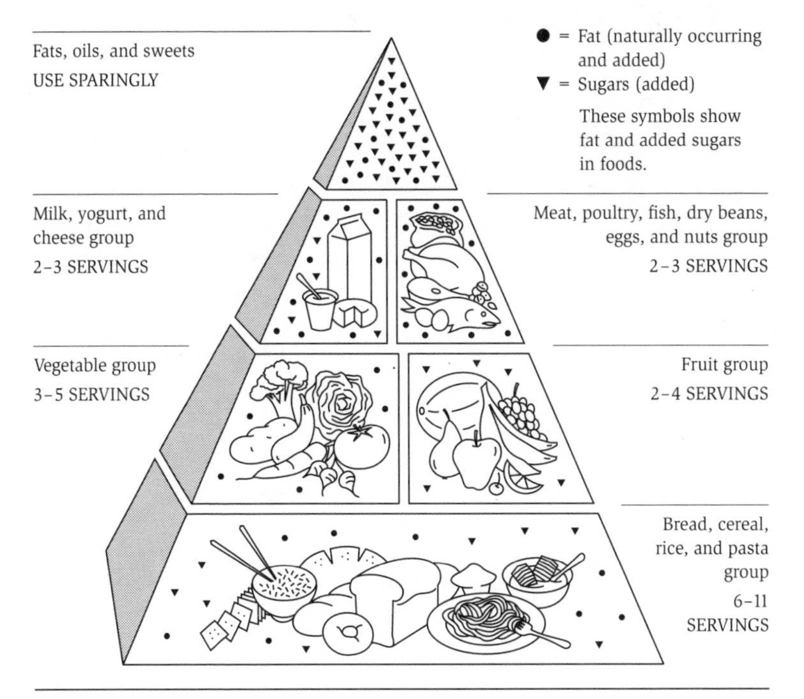

FIGURE 4-1. A daily food guide visualized with most portions coming from grains and the least from fats and sweets.

and sweets should be consumed in limited amounts, these items are grouped in a small section at the top of the pyramid. Alcoholic beverages are also part of this group. Fats, sweets, and alcohol are often called empty calories because they are high in calories but low in most nutrients.

The number of calories that the Food Guide Pyramid provides will vary, depending on the selection of foods within the groups and the number of servings eaten. The minimum number of servings from the Food Guide Pyramid provides about 1,600 calories if you choose low-fat, lean foods from the five groups and use items from the fats and sweets group sparingly. Eating the minimum number of servings from the pyramid will promote body fat loss for most people while providing adequate nutrients.

Consuming the maximum number of servings (with a limited use of fats and sweets) provides about 2,800 calories. If you need more calories, you can eat a greater number of servings from the food groups by eating between-meal snacks. There's no harm in eating some high-carbohydrate empty calories once you've met your nutrient needs, but you can't go wrong adding extra servings of grain products, fruit, and vegetables (see the serving size guidelines in Table 4-1).

Developing a High-Carbohydrate Diet

A practical high-carbohydrate diet can also be created by using the Food Exchange System shown in Table 4-2 on pp. 40–41. The exchange lists are the basis of a meal planning system developed by the American Dietetic Association and the American Diabetes Association.

TABLE 4-1
HOW MANY SERVINGS DO YOU NEED EACH DAY?

CALORIE LEVEL*	WOMEN AND SOME OLDER ADULTS	CHILDREN, TEEN GIRLS, ACTIVE WOMEN, MOST MEN	TEEN BOYS AND ACTIVE MEN
	ABOUT 1,600	ABOUT 2,200	ABOUT 2,800
Bread Group	6	9	11
Vegetable Group	3	4	5
Fruit Group	2	3	4
Milk Group	2–3**	2–3**	2–3**
Meat Group	2	2	3
Total ounces per day	5	6	7

*These are the calorie levels if you choose low-fat, lean foods from the 5 major food groups and use foods from the fats, oils, and sweets group sparingly.
**Women who are pregnant or breastfeeding, teenagers, and young adults to age 24 need 3 servings.

SOURCE: U.S. Department of Agriculture and the U.S. Department of Health and Human Services.

There are six food planning exchange lists: grain, vegetables, fruit, meat, milk, and fat. Each one lists foods that have about the same number of carbohydrate, protein, fat, and calories. Any food on a list can be exchanged or traded for any other food on the same list.

These food exchange lists can be used to plan diets that provide 1,500 to 4,000 calories a day while supplying about 60% carbohydrate, 15% protein, and less than 25% fat (see Table 4-3 on p. 41). As a general guide, starchy foods and fruit provide the highest amount of carbohydrate (15 gram) per serving. Milk is the next highest source, providing 12 grams per serving. And vegetables provide 5 grams per serving. To keep your intake of fat low, choose low-fat or

TABLE 4-2
FOOD GROUP EXCHANGES

STARCH/BREAD/GRAINS (80 CALORIES)
15 grams carbohydrate; 3 grams protein; 0 grams fat
1/2 cup pasta, barley, cooked cereal
1/3 cup rice or dried cooked peas/beans
1/2 cup corn, peas, winter squash
1 small (3 oz.) baked potato
4–6 crackers
1 slice bread or 6″ tortilla
1/2 bagel, English muffin, pita
3/4 cup dry flaked cereal
3 cups popcorn, no oil or butter
3/4 oz. pretzels

MEAT AND MEAT ALTERNATIVES (55–100 CALORIES)
0 grams carbohydrate; 7 grams protein; 3–8 grams fat
1 oz. poultry, fish, beef, pork, lamb, etc.
1/4 cup tuna, salmon, cottage cheese
2 tbsp. peanut butter
1 egg
1 oz. cheese
tofu (2 1/2″ × 2 3/4″ × 1″)

VEGETABLES (25 CALORIES)
5 grams carbohydrate; 2 grams protein; 0 grams fat
1/2 cup cooked vegetables
1 cup raw vegetables
1/2 cup tomato or vegetable juice

MILK (90–150 CALORIES)
12 grams carbohydrate; 8 grams protein; 0–5 grams fat
1 cup milk: nonfat, low-fat, 1%, whole
1 cup yogurt: nonfat, low-fat, 1%, whole

TABLE 4-2 *(continued)*

FRUIT (60 CALORIES)
15 grams carbohydrate; 0 grams protein; 0 grams fat
1 medium fresh fruit
1 cup berries or melon
1/2 cup canned fruit (without sugar)
1/2 cup fruit juice
1/4 cup dried fruit

FAT (45 CALORIES)
0 grams carbohydrate; 0 grams protein; 5 grams fat
1 tsp. margarine, oil, butter, mayonnaise
2 tsp. diet margarine, diet mayonnaise
1 tbsp. salad dressing, cream cheese, cream, nuts
2 tbsp. diet salad dressing, sour cream
1 slice bacon

TABLE 4-3
TRAINING DIET MEAL PLANS

	NUMBER OF EXCHANGES					
	CALORIE LEVEL					
FOOD GROUP	1,500	2,000	2,500	3,000	3,500	4,000
Milk	3	3	4	4	4	4
Meat	5	5	5	5	6	6
Fruit	5	6	7	9	10	12
Vegetable	3	3	3	5	6	7
Grain	7	11	16	18	20	24
Fat	2	3	5	6	8	10

nonfat foods from the milk and meat lists. As noted, sugary foods such as cookies, cake, pie, soft drinks, and candy can supply additional carbohydrate but are low in most other nutrients.

Complex Carbohydrates and Sugar

Complex carbohydrates (starch) and sugar are grouped together as carbohydrates because they have a chemical similarity. All carbohydrates are made up of one or more simple sugars, the three most common being glucose, fructose, and galactose. The simple sugar glucose connected to fructose forms sucrose, or table sugar. When more than two glucose molecules are connected, they become a complex carbohydrate. Complex carbohydrates contain from 300 to 1,000 or more glucose units linked together. Our body uses both the sugars and starches for energy.

Although there appear to be no differences in glycogen storage between complex carbohydrates and refined carbohydrates, a high-performance diet emphasizes complex carbohydrates. Foods high in complex carbohydrates such as bread, cereal, rice, beans, pasta, and vegetables also supply other nutrients such as vitamins, minerals, protein, and fiber. Sweet foods that are high in sugar (e.g., candy bars, doughnuts, and cookies) supply carbohydrate, but they also contain a high amount of fat and only insignificant amounts of vitamins and minerals.

Fruit contains the sweetest of all simple sugars—fructose. Because fruit is mostly water, its sugar and calorie content are relatively low. Like starchy foods, most fruits are rich in nutrients and virtually fat free.

Commercial Carbohydrate Supplements

Some people train so heavily that they have difficulty eating enough food to meet their carbohydrate needs. This can happen for several reasons.

Often the stress of hard training can decrease appetite, resulting in reduced consumption of carbohydrate and calories. Eating a large volume of food can also cause gastrointestinal discomfort and interfere with training. And some people spend so much time training that there aren't many rest hours available for replenishment.

People who have problems consuming enough carbohydrate can use a commercial high-carbohydrate supplement (see Table 4-4 on p. 44). These products do not replace regular food but are designed to supply supplemental calories and carbohydrate when needed. If you can consume an adequate amount of food, these products are unnecessary.

High-carbohydrate supplements should be consumed before or after exercise, either with meals or between meals. They are too concentrated in carbohydrate to be used as fluid replacement drinks during exercise.

Nutrition Counseling

Beware of self-proclaimed nutrition "experts" who promote questionable foods, supplements, and fad diets. The title *nutritionist* can be used by anyone, regardless of training. Under the heading *nutritionist,* you have more than a 50% chance of finding a person with phony credentials or someone who delivers false information. If you want individual

TABLE 4-4
HIGH-CARBOHYDRATE BEVERAGES

BEVERAGE	FLAVORS	CARBO-HYDRATE INGREDIENT	CARBOHYDRATE % (CONCENTRATION) 12-OZ. SERVING	CARBO-HYDRATE	SODIUM
GatorLode® High Carbohydrate Loading and Recovery Drink The Gatorade Company	Lemon, citrus, banana	Maltodextrin, glucose	20	70	95
Carboplex® Unipro, Inc.	Plain	Maltodextrin	24	82	0
Carbo Power® Nature's Best Food Supplements	Lemonade, strawberry, fruit punch, orange, grape, tea	Maltodextrin, high-fructose corn syrup	18	64	76
Ultra Fuel® Twin Labs	Lemon, lime, grape, fruit punch, orange	Maltodextrin, glucose, fructose	21	75	0
ProOptibol® 105 Next Nutrition	Wild berry	Glucose, fructose	19	66	0
Cybergenics Cybercharge® L & S Research Corp.	Lemon, lime, grape	Glucose, polymers, fructose	21	75	15
Carbo Fire® Weider Health & Fitness	Tropical punch, orange	Glucose, polymers, fructose	24	83	60

nutrition counseling, consult a registered dietitian (credentials abbreviated R.D.).

A registered dietitian is a health care professional who is educated in nutrition and food science. For a person to become an R.D., the American Dietetic Association (ADA) requires specific course work from an accredited university (minimum of a bachelor of science degree), completion of a nutrition internship at an approved hospital, and a passing score on a national certification exam. Registered dietitians are required to continue their professional education by attending scientific meetings or by writing scientific papers and giving lectures to colleagues.

You can find an R.D. by requesting a referral from your physician, or by contacting the nutrition department of a hospital, clinic, or community health agency. You can also look in the phone book under dietitians, nutritionists, and weight control; remember to look for the initials R.D. behind the name.

There are registered dietitians who specialize in sports nutrition. They usually belong to the Sports, Cardiovascular, and Wellness Nutrition Group (abbreviated SCAN) of the American Dietetic Association. You can be referred to SCAN members in your geographic area by calling the American Dietetic Association at 1-800-366-1655.

5

Carbohydrate Loading

Filling Your Tank with High-Octane Fuel

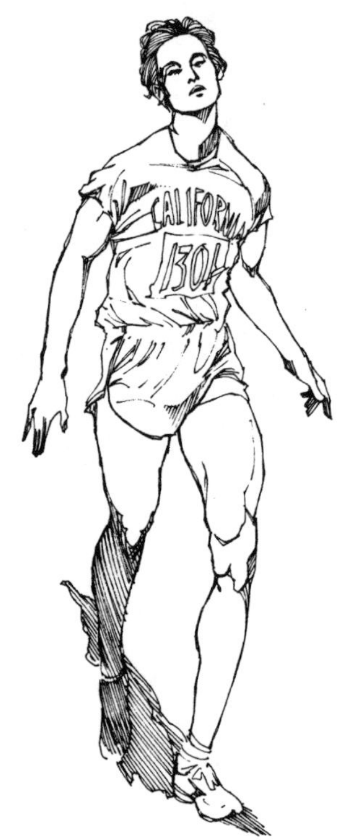

I thought muscle glycogen depletion was a crackpot theory until I experienced it.

I was running my third marathon. I had averaged 8-minute miles all the way out and passed the 15 and 18 mile markers with no problems—feeling fine.

At the 20th mile I felt weak and had problems lifting my legs. It took a concerted effort to run.

By the 21st mile, 2 hours and 40 minutes out, that was it. I couldn't run. There was nothing left. I felt excruciating pain in my thighs. Everything hurt. Walking hurt, but it was possible. I walked the last 5 miles. Each time I tried to run, I couldn't lift my legs. Even to try was extremely painful. Later, after the fact, I thought I had just lacked will power.

In my next marathon, though, I encountered the same situation. After about 3 hours, I just couldn't run slowly enough. Couldn't even shuffle. I walked in again.

After that I became a firm believer in "the wall."

As originally developed, the glycogen-loading regimen was difficult to follow. Athletes either gave up on the regimen or were too intimidated to try it. The revised diet involves no hardship and is just as effective. However, you need to follow basic ground rules to get the performance benefit.

The Wall

When your muscle glycogen stores drop to critically low levels (the point of glycogen depletion), high-intensity exercise cannot be maintained. In practical terms, you are exhausted and must either stop exercising or drastically reduce your pace. Marathon runners frequently refer to muscle glycogen depletion as "hitting the wall." The wall usually occurs at around the 20-mile mark and running becomes virtually impossible for many athletes.

Glycogen Stores and Endurance

An obvious way to improve your endurance (when you're exercising longer than 90 minutes) is to increase your muscle glycogen stores. The higher your pre-exercise muscle glycogen level, the greater will be your endurance potential. This is the rationale behind carbohydrate loading. When done properly, carbohydrate loading can increase your muscle glycogen stores by 50% to 100%.

Let's take a practical look at what this means. If you eat a normal American diet (about 4 to 5 grams per kilogram of body weight daily), you can exercise hard (at 75% of your $\dot{V}O_{2max}$) for 1 1/2 to 2 hours before muscle glycogen depletion. After following the carbohydrate-loading regimen (10 grams of carbohydrate per kilogram of body weight daily with tapered training), you can exercise at the same intensity for 3 hours. Carbohydrate loading can buy you an additional hour or more of high-intensity exercise per day.

Carbohydrate loading is most effective when you follow a specific week-long diet and exercise plan.

The Original Diet

As originally practiced, carbohydrate loading was hard to follow because of the extreme diet shifts during the last week of training. Seven days before competition, you would exercise hard for 90 minutes, specifically working the muscles you would use in your event. You would taper training for the next 3 days and eat a low-carbohydrate diet (below 40% carbohydrate). The purpose of the low-carbohydrate diet was to further lower your muscle glycogen levels. For the 3 days immediately prior to competition, you would switch to a carbohydrate-rich diet (at least 70% carbohydrate) and finally rest. The depleted muscles would then gobble up glycogen to the point of maximum storage. For many years, this week-long sequence was considered the best way to ensure maximum glycogen storage.

However, the low-carbohydrate diet component of the old technique caused many people to quit the regimen—

or avoid it altogether. Three days on a low-carbohydrate diet can cause low blood sugar (hypoglycemia) and increased blood acids from fat breakdown (ketosis), with associated nausea, fatigue, dizziness, and irritability. Attempting to train with such abnormally low muscle glycogen stores was a sheer test of will power. Also, the abrupt switching from a low- to a high-carbohydrate diet proved to be too cumbersome for many athletes, and they couldn't stick with the week-long sequence.

The Revised Diet

A revised version of carbohydrate loading eliminates many of the problems associated with the classical routine (see Table 5-1). On the sixth day before the event, you exercise hard (70% to 75% $\dot{V}O_{2max}$) for 90 minutes. On the fifth and fourth days before the event, decrease your training to 40 minutes (still at 70% to 75% $\dot{V}O_{2max}$). During the first 3 days, you eat a normal diet providing about 5 grams of carbohydrate per kilogram of body weight per day (about 50% carbohydrate). On the third and second day before the event, you reduce your training to 20 minutes. On the day before the event, you rest. During the last 3 days, you eat a high-carbohydrate diet providing 10 grams of carbohydrate per kilogram of body weight per day (about 70% carbohydrate).

This modified sequence produces muscle glycogen levels equal to those provided by the classic regimen. However, the new routine eliminates the misery created by the low-carbohydrate diet and requires only one major dietary change—switching from an average American diet

TABLE 5-1
TRAINING AND DIET REGIMEN FOR GLYCOGEN LOADING

DAY	TRAINING	EATING	
1	90 min • 70–75% $\dot{V}O_{2max}$	50% carbohydrate	5 gm/kg
2	40 min • 70–75% $\dot{V}O_{2max}$	50% carbohydrate	5 gm/kg
3	40 min • 70–75% $\dot{V}O_{2max}$	50% carbohydrate	5 gm/kg
4	20 min • 70–75% $\dot{V}O_{2max}$	70% carbohydrate	10 gm/kg
5	20 min • 70–75% $\dot{V}O_{2max}$	70% carbohydrate	10 gm/kg
6	Rest	70% carbohydrate	10 gm/kg
7	Event	Event	

to a high-carbohydrate diet (the same diet you eat during heavy training).

Why Do Your Muscles Store More Glycogen?

The classic carbohydrate-loading technique used a low-carbohydrate diet in the belief that you had to absolutely deplete your glycogen stores to achieve maximum glycogen storage. Now we know that endurance training is the primary stimulus for increased muscle glycogen synthesis. Endurance training increases the activity of glycogen synthase—the enzyme responsible for glycogen storage. Tapering your training and eating a high-carbohydrate diet allows the muscles to store more glycogen.

Because exercise is the primary stimulus for greater

muscle glycogen storage, you need to be endurance trained or carbohydrate loading won't work. If you're unfit and try carbohydrate loading, your muscles won't store more than their usual amount of glycogen. Even without carbohydrate loading, rested elite marathoners have muscle glycogen levels twice as high as normal and equal to the levels found in the carbohydrate-loaded muscle of an average athlete. Elite endurance athletes may not benefit as much from the carbohydrate-loading technique.

Selecting Food

When you eat an average American diet, you consume about 250 to 350 grams of carbohydrate per day, and get about 50% of your calories from carbohydrate. To get a high-carbohydrate diet of 10 grams per kilogram of body weight daily (about 70% of calories), most athletes need to consume at least 500 to 600 grams of carbohydrate.

To obtain a high-carbohydrate diet, you will need to eat more carbohydrate-rich foods than you eat during training. Breads, pasta, cereal, beans, rice, potatoes, corn, pancakes, and other starchy foods and fruit are the primary sources of carbohydrate. Other good sources include milk, yogurt, and vegetables. Ice milk and milkshakes, and high-sugar foods such as cakes, cookies, pies, soft drinks, and candy are also high in carbohydrate. Two sample menus are shown in Tables 5-2 and 5-3.

If you have difficulty obtaining enough carbohydrate, you can consider taking a high-carbohydrate supplement (see Table 4-4 on p. 44). For example, 24 ounces of

GatorLode® provides 140 grams of carbohydrate, and 24 ounces of Carboplex® provides 164 grams of carbohydrate.

Don't ignore your nutritional needs during carbohydrate loading. As followed by some athletes, the diet can be deficient in the vitamins and minerals necessary for peak performance and good health.

When you eat only a few carbohydrate sources or consume large amounts of refined carbohydrates, your diet can easily be deficient. Lots of sweets can also result in gastrointestinal distress in the form of cramps, nausea, diarrhea, and bloating. You should emphasize complex carbohydrates over sweets for carbohydrate loading (as well as good health in general), because they provide nutrients with their calories.

Exercise and Glycogen Stores

You should keep several things in mind when you carbohydrate load. First, the exercise to deplete your glycogen stores must be the same as your own competitive event, because glycogen stores are specific to the muscle groups used. For example, a cyclist needs to deplete his stores by cycling rather than by running.

Second, it is essential that you decrease your training the 3 days prior to competition. Too much exercise during this period will use up too much of your stored glycogen and defeat the purpose of the entire process. This final 3 days, when you taper and eat a high-carbohydrate diet, is the real loading phase of the regimen.

Table 5-2
Sample Glycogen Loading Menu 1

Breakfast	
1 cup orange juice	
1 cup oatmeal, with	
1 banana	
1 cup low-fat milk	
1 slices wheat bread, with	
1 tsp. margarine	
Lunch	**Snack**
2 slices rye bread	8 graham crackers
3 oz. turkey	1 cup low-fat milk
1 oz. mozzarella cheese, with lettuce, tomato, mustard	1 apple
1 tsp. mayonnaise	
1 cup apple juice	
1 orange	
1 cup lemon sherbet	
Dinner	**Snack**
2 cups spaghetti	6 cups popcorn, air popped
2/3 cup tomato sauce, with mushrooms	
2 tbsp. Parmesan cheese	
4 slices French bread	
2 tsp. margarine	
1/2 cup broccoli	
1/2 cup ice cream, with	
3/4 cup strawberries	

Sample menu contains approximately 3,000 calories: 518 grams of carbohydrate.

TABLE 5-3
SAMPLE GLYCOGEN LOADING MENU 2

BREAKFAST	SNACK
2 cups corn flakes 1 cup nonfat milk 2 cups orange juice (frozen) 3 slices cracked wheat bread 3 tsp. jelly	2 large bananas
LUNCH	**SNACK**
6 slices cracked wheat bread 3 oz. turkey 3 oz. low-fat American cheese 2 cups apple juice	2 almond granola bars
DINNER	**SNACK**
3 cups spaghetti, with marinara sauce 2 medium rolls 2 tbsp. margarine 1 cup green beans 1 cup nonfat milk 2 large oranges	2 large apples

Sample menu contains approximately 4,000 calories: 607 grams of carbohydrate.

Limitations

Carbohydrate loading has several side effects that may make it inappropriate for some people. For each gram of glycogen stored, additional water is stored. Some people note a feeling of stiffness and heaviness associated with the increased glycogen storage. Once you start exercising, however, these sensations will work out.

If you have heart disease, diabetes, and/or high blood triglycerides, you may have problems if you carbohydrate load. When in doubt, check with your doctor before attempting this regimen.

Remember that carbohydrate loading will help only for continuous exercise lasting more than 90 minutes. Greater than usual muscle glycogen stores won't enable you to exercise harder during shorter duration exercise. In fact, the stiffness and heaviness that result from increased glycogen stores can hurt your performance during shorter competitions such as a 10K run.

Keep in mind that carbohydrate loading enables you to maintain high-intensity exercise longer, but will not affect your pace for the first hour of exercise. You won't be able to go out faster, but you will be able to maintain your pace longer.

6

Fat

Friend or Foe?

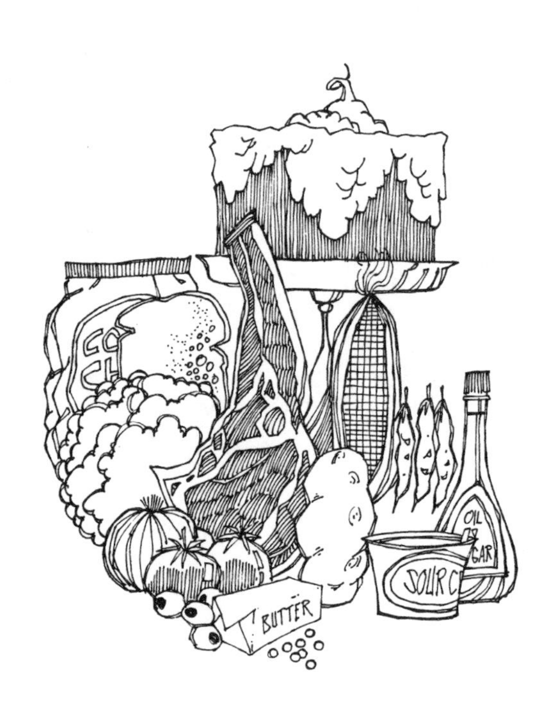

Wednesday night I visited a friend who planned to run a marathon on Saturday. He was cooking a dinner that consisted of steak, a baked potato with sour cream, a vegetable smothered in butter, a salad with lots of dressing, and bread. For dessert, he planned cake. While he was cooking, he ate half a bag of corn chips.

"What are you getting ready for?" I asked him.

"I'm carbohydrate loading," he replied.

"No, you're not," I said. "You're fat loading."

FAT IS DEFINITELY OUT OF FASHION. We fight fat to look good, and we are increasingly aware of the health risks of high-fat diets. But fat burning plays a positive role in endurance exercise. In fact, a major benefit of endurance training is the increased ability to use fat for energy.

The Importance of Fat as Fuel

The importance of being able to use fat for fuel can be illustrated by comparing elite and average marathon runners. Most average marathon runners dread the experience of hitting the wall. When elite runners have been questioned, however, many say they don't worry about it. Why the difference?

As noted in the previous chapter, "hitting the wall" is synonymous with muscle glycogen depletion, which occurs within 90 to 120 minutes of exercise at 75% $\dot{V}O_{2max}$. The elite marathoner escapes the wall primarily because he completes the race before his glycogen stores are depleted. His exceptionally high $\dot{V}O_{2max}$ and lactate threshold both enable him to run marathons in approximately 2 hours. The elite marathoner also does not hit the wall because he uses muscle glycogen at a slower rate.

Endurance training increases your utilization of fat as fuel. This increased fat-burning ability spares muscle glycogen. Because muscle glycogen depletion limits endurance, slowing your rate of glycogen depletion will improve your performance in endurance events.

Whereas our total glycogen stores (in muscle and liver) amount to only about 2,000 calories, every pound of fat supplies 3,500 calories. Fat is the major fuel for light- to moderate-intensity exercise (up to 60% of $\dot{V}O_{2max}$).

Even though fat makes significant energy contributions during prolonged endurance exercise, you shouldn't attempt to store fat as you would glycogen. All of us store more fat than we ever need, and excess body fat impairs athletic performance. Also, if you eat more fat, you'll eat less carbohydrate. Muscle glycogen stores cannot be adequately maintained on a high-fat diet.

Fat in the Diet

Fats, or lipids, are the most concentrated source of food energy. One gram of fat supplies about nine calories, compared to the four calories per gram supplied by carbohydrate and protein. Fat is the body's only source of a fatty acid called linoleic acid that is essential for growth and healthy skin and hair. Fat insulates and protects the body's organs against trauma and exposure to cold. Fats make our food taste better and keep us from getting hungry for a longer period of time between meals. Fats are also involved in the absorption and transport of the fat-soluble vitamins.

Fats are the source of fatty acids, which are divided into two categories—saturated and unsaturated (including polyunsaturated and monounsaturated fatty acids). These fatty acids differ from each other chemically because of the nature of the bond between carbon and hydrogen atoms.

As a general rule, saturated fat (e.g., butter and lard) is solid at room temperature and is derived mainly from animal sources. Unsaturated fat (e.g., safflower, canola, and corn oil) is liquid at room temperature and found mainly in plant sources. Palm and coconut oils are exceptions; they are highly saturated vegetable fats.

The average American diet supplies 37% of the calories from fat. All evidence suggests that this is too much—for endurance athletes as well as sedentary people. Fat amounts this high increase your risk of developing heart disease (our nation's number one killer), stroke, and certain cancers. A high-fat diet also contributes to obesity, which is associated with a wide range of health problems.

Athletes, like all Americans, should consume no more than 30% of their total calories from fat and limit dietary cholesterol to 300 milligrams per day. Because saturated fat increases the cholesterol level in the blood, it should provide no more than 10% of total calories. An elevated blood cholesterol level is a major risk factor for heart disease, as are smoking, high blood pressure, and inactivity.

Cutting Down on Fat Intake

You can lower your fat intake by cutting down on both hidden and visible sources of fat. Fat is hidden in dairy products, meat, eggs, nuts, and fried foods. Be aware of the hidden fat in foods such as ice cream, cheese, french fries, chips, granola, cold cuts, bacon, nuts, hamburger, and baked goods (cookies, pies, cakes, and pastries). Visible dietary sources of fat include margarine, butter, cream, mayonnaise, oil, salad dressing, gravies, sauces, sour cream, and cream cheese.

Your intake of total fat, saturated fat, and cholesterol can be reduced by choosing lean meat, poultry, and fish. Try to eat less high-fat processed meat such as bologna, bacon, salami, and hot dogs. Removing the skin from poultry and trimming visible fat from meat also cuts down on fat. The Dietary Guidelines for Americans recommend limiting the consumption of meat, poultry, and fish to about 6 ounces per day.

The butterfat found in butter, cheese, chocolate, ice cream, and whole milk can also be limited to reduce your intake of total fat, saturated fat, and cholesterol. Substitute nonfat and low-fat dairy products such as 1% fat milk and yogurt, ice milk, and low-fat cheese for high-fat dairy products. The Dietary Guidelines for Americans recommend consuming two to three servings of dairy products each day.

Oils with high percentages of unsaturated fat (canola, corn, olive, and soy oil and their derivative margarines) should be substituted for saturated fats such as butter, lard, shortening, and bacon grease. When oil and margarine are substituted for butter, remember that they are still high in fat and calories and should be used sparingly. Nonfat substitutes for salad dressing and sour cream can replace the regular higher fat versions.

Choose cooking methods that require little or no fat. These include steaming, baking, broiling, grilling, poaching, or stir-frying in small amounts of unsaturated vegetable oil. Foods can be microwaved or cooked in pans that have been sprayed with nonstick products to reduce added fat. Try to limit fried foods, especially when saturated fat is used.

Although nonfat and low-fat bakery goods and frozen dairy products contain little or no fat, they do contain calories. Remember to check the food label; fat free does not mean calorie free. These products can be loaded with extra sugar to improve taste.

Increasing Ability to Use Fat

Although there is no advantage to excess body fat stores or a high-fat diet, there is an advantage in increasing the body's utilization of fat. The ability to use fat will spare muscle glycogen and improve endurance.

Your $\dot{V}O_{2max}$ and lactate threshold have a positive effect on the contribution of fat during endurance exercise. In general, the higher your $\dot{V}O_{2max}$ and lactate threshold, the greater will be your ability to use fat.

Endurance training also causes several major adaptations in the muscles that increase fat utilization. First, endurance training increases the number of capillaries in the trained muscles, so that the muscles receive more blood and oxygen. Second, endurance training increases the activity of the specific muscle enzymes that are responsible for burning fat.

If you want to increase your capacity for fat utilization, make sure your workouts last at least an hour. The longer they are, the better (remember that it takes at least 20 minutes for fat utilization to kick in). Also, keep your intensity at around 60% of $\dot{V}O_{2max}$. If your workout is too intense (over 70% of $\dot{V}O_{2max}$), your muscles will shift from fat toward glycogen utilization.

High-intensity workouts (e.g., with interval training) are done to increase speed, not to improve fat utilization. You may also increase your utilization of fat by consuming caffeine prior to exercise. We discuss the pros and cons of caffeine in Chapter 11.

Fat Loading

High-fat diets are sometimes promoted to improve performance in endurance events. The claim is that "fat loading" enables you to burn fat, rather than glycogen, as your major fuel source. Because fat stores are plentiful and glycogen stores are limited, fat loading supposedly enhances endurance.

Cyclists who ate a high-fat diet (85% of calories) for 1 month used three times less muscle glycogen and four times less blood glucose during exercise at 63% of $\dot{V}O_{2max}$. Their utilization of fat rose to make up the difference.

Don't buy that steak yet, though. First, the high-fat diet did not improve performance compared to a diet containing 50% carbohydrate. Second, the drawbacks of high-fat diets outweigh any potential benefits. Such diets need medical supervision because they have been associated with sudden death and heart rhythm disturbances, resulting from loss of protein in the heart and potassium depletion. The cyclists were constantly monitored for lost electrolytes, and these were replaced throughout the study.

Although the cyclists trained heavily, their blood

cholesterol levels increased while they were on the high-fat diet. As exercise by itself does not fully protect someone against heart disease, eating a high-fat diet for a prolonged period may contribute to an increased risk that an individual will develop cardiac problems.

A high-fat diet is also hard to digest, and this is one of the reasons that fat should be limited in the pre-exercise meal. The high-fat meals in this study consisted of butter, cheese, cream, ground or marbled beef, and tuna with dollops of mayonnaise. Such a diet isn't palatable and lacks the variety needed for optimum nutrient intake.

Adaptation to a high-fat diet takes at least 2 weeks. Exercise during this time will be difficult and unpleasant, because of low glycogen stores. Even when adaptation is complete, your ability to exercise hard (70% or more of $\dot{V}O_{2max}$) may be impaired. Remember: In many events, you're competing at 70% or more of your $\dot{V}O_{2max}$.

The study can be criticized on several fronts. It did not compare a high-carbohydrate diet (8 to 10 grams per kilogram of body weight, or 65% to 70% of calories) to the high-fat diet. A high-carbohydrate diet would provide higher glycogen stores than the 50% carbohydrate diet used in the study, and thus would result in a longer cycling time to exhaustion.

Also, the cyclists exercised to exhaustion at an exercise intensity low enough (63% of $\dot{V}O_{2max}$) to be fueled by fat and not limited by muscle glycogen depletion. If these tests had been conducted at an exercise intensity known to be limited by muscle glycogen depletion (70% or more of $\dot{V}O_{2max}$), impaired endurance would be expected.

So a high-fat diet may not buy you any endurance advantage after all. Why feel lousy for 4 weeks while trying to adjust to a high-fat diet when you can feel good and perform well (without any adaptation) on a high-carbohydrate diet?

Your ability to burn fat is increased far more effectively by endurance training than by eating a high-fat diet. In any case, the harmful health effects of high-fat diets make them too risky for endurance athletes.

7

Protein

The Great American Protein Myth

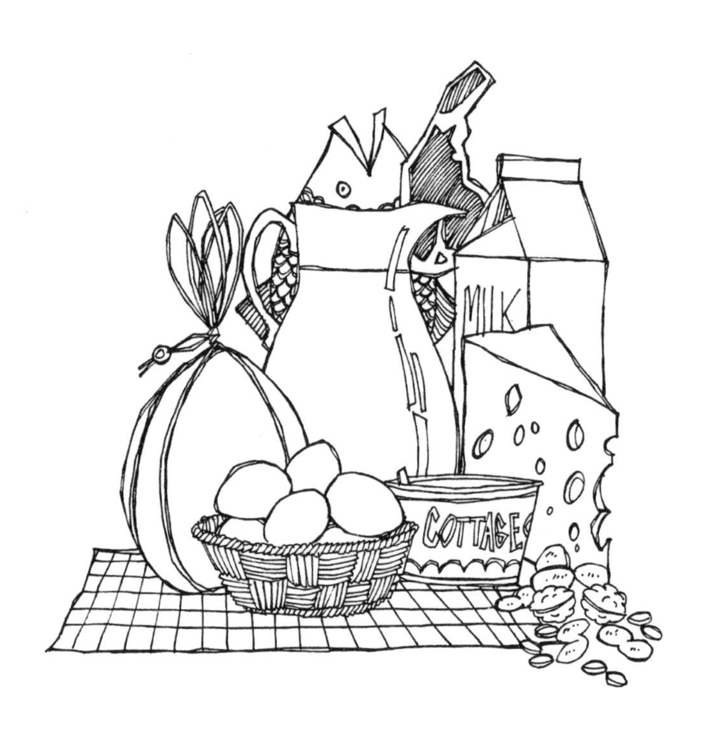

A friend of mine in her late 20s had been running for 10 years. She felt good during runs, but thought she needed to lose weight, so she went on a diet. While on the diet, she complained that she had no energy, to the point that at times she couldn't run at all.

"What's the diet?" I asked her.

For breakfast she had an egg; at lunch she drank a protein supplement with milk; and for dinner she ate cottage cheese, a hamburger patty, and a piece of bread.

I asked her what she really wanted to eat.

"Sweets," she said. "I want sweets."

I told her to come off the diet and eat more bread, fruits and vegetables, and starchy foods in general. She kept the level of calories she was eating the same. She lost her craving for sweets, had plenty of energy, and felt fine.

If this woman couldn't find the energy to run, she must have felt very bad. She later told me that it had been easier to run while she was pregnant than it had been to run during that diet. She was eating so much protein that she couldn't maintain her glycogen stores. She didn't get enough carbohydrates to perform well.

AMERICANS HAVE BEEN SOLD on the idea that protein is the "good guy." In fact, protein is essential for health, and vigorous exercise does place special demands on protein needs. However, protein is no more essential than other nutrients. It is a poor energy source, and too much can be expensive and potentially detrimental. A balanced diet supplies more than enough for any athlete.

Protein in the Diet

Protein is a major structural component of all body tissues and is required for tissue growth and repair. Proteins are necessary components of hormones, enzymes, and blood plasma transport systems.

The proteins in both animal and plant foods are composed of structural units called amino acids. Of the more than 20 amino acids that have been identified, nine must be provided by our diet and are called essential amino acids. Meat, fish, dairy products, eggs, and poultry contain all nine essential amino acids and are called complete proteins. Vegetable proteins, such as beans and grains, are called incomplete proteins because they do not supply all the essential amino acids.

The body can make complete proteins if a variety of plant foods—beans, grains, vegetables, fruits, nuts, and seeds—and sufficient calories are eaten during the day. Vegetarians need not worry about combining specific foods within a meal as the old "complementary protein" theory advised. Well-balanced vegetarian diets may even decrease the risk of heart disease and cancer because they are lower in fat and higher in complex carbohydrates than the average American diet.

Protein Needs and Exercise

Athletes do need more protein than sedentary people. Exercise may promote a loss of muscle protein through reduced protein synthesis and increased protein breakdown. The hormonal changes that occur during exercise—increased epinephrine and decreased insulin levels—may be responsible for these effects of exercise on protein metabolism.

Exercise may also promote body protein loss in other ways. Protein has been found in the urine of runners after marathons and may also be lost in sweat.

Regular physical training tends to reduce muscle protein breakdown and protein loss from the body. Although some protein breakdown may predominate during exercise, protein buildup is enhanced in the recovery period that follows. Regular exercise seems to increase the effectiveness of the protein synthesis that occurs during recovery.

Protein as Fuel

As discussed in Chapter 3, several factors influence what the muscles use as fuel during exercise. The two most important of these are the duration of exercise and the carbohydrate content of the diet.

When muscle glycogen stores are low, due to prolonged exercise or a low-carbohydrate diet, protein may contribute as much as 15% of the energy needed for exercise. However, when muscle glycogen stores are high, the contribution of protein for energy is no more than about 5%. You will also use more protein for fuel when you don't eat enough calories. Consuming adequate calories in a high-carbohydrate diet during repeated days of heavy training helps to maintain muscle glycogen stores and reduces the use of protein as fuel.

Protein Requirements

The Recommended Dietary Allowance (RDA) of protein for sedentary adults is 0.8 gram per kilogram of body weight. Endurance athletes need 50% to 75% more protein than the adult RDA. This means that you require 1.2 grams per kilogram of body weight daily and may benefit by consuming 1.4 grams per kilogram during prolonged endurance exercise.

An increased protein intake appears to be more important during the early stages of your training than later in the training program. You initially need more protein to support increases in the aerobic enzymes (proteins) in the muscle and to build red blood cells and myoglobin (an oxygen carrier in the muscle similar to hemoglobin).

You can obtain 1.2 to 1.4 grams of protein per kilogram of body weight when your diet provides 12% to 15% of calories as protein. This amount of protein is consistent with the dietary recommendations for athletes—60% to 70% carbohydrate, 12% to 15% protein, and 20% to 30% fat.

These protein guidelines assume that you are consuming enough calories. You need more protein when you don't eat enough calories (due to heavy training), or when you reduce your caloric intake to lower your body weight or body fat. Your protein requirement increases because the protein is used for energy rather than for muscle growth and repair.

When you eat enough to meet your calorie needs, getting enough protein is easy. The average sedentary American consumes about 100 grams of protein per day for a total protein intake of about 1.4 grams per kilogram of body weight, or 16% of total calories. About 70% of this protein comes from animal sources, which contain all the essential amino acids.

Athletes consume more protein when their caloric intake increases as a result of training. For example, let's say that a sedentary 70-kilogram man decides to train for a marathon. Over a period of time, his daily caloric intake gradually increases from 2,500 to 3,500 calories. His protein intake would increase from 94 to 131 grams per day if 15% of his calories came from protein. His daily protein intake relative to body weight would increase from 1.3 grams per kilogram to 1.8 grams per kilogram, which would be more than adequate.

Good sources of complete proteins are meat, poultry, fish, dairy products, and eggs. An ounce of meat, poultry, or cheese, or one egg supplies about 7 grams of protein containing all the essential amino acids. Milk and yogurt are also excellent complete protein sources, with 8 ounces supplying 8 grams of protein. To reduce dietary fat, try to emphasize lean meat, chicken or turkey without the skin, and nonfat or 1% fat dairy products.

Amino Acid Supplements

Amino acid supplements are popular among athletes such as body builders and weight lifters who are trying to "bulk up." Proponents of amino acid supplements claim that certain amino acids increase muscle mass and decrease body fat.

Arginine and ornithine are particular supplement favorites as they supposedly stimulate the secretion of growth hormone, thereby increasing muscle mass and decreasing body fat. Consuming large amounts of these amino acids may cause a temporary rise in growth hormone levels, but there is no proof that this rise increases muscle mass or reduces body fat. Endurance training and weight lifting both significantly increase growth hormone levels. Combining amino acid supplements with exercise does not increase growth hormone levels above those seen with exercise.

Athletes may hear that only a small amount of the amino acids in foods are digested and absorbed. This is not correct. The truth is that about 95% to 99% of the amino acids from animal sources and about 90% of the amino acids from vegetable sources are digested and utilized by the body.

Athletes may also be told that amino acids do not need to be digested before absorption and so replenish the body's proteins faster than the amino acids from high-protein foods. There is no evidence that more rapid absorption is beneficial; it takes hours, not minutes, to rebuild muscle proteins damaged during intense exercise.

A further claim for amino acid supplements is that they provide all the amino acids provided by food but are less taxing to the body's digestive system. Actually, the body quite readily produces an array of digestive enzymes that systematically break down the protein in food to amino acids before absorption.

Amino acid supplements usually contain only 200 to 500 milligrams of amino acids per capsule. On the other hand, 1 ounce of beef, chicken, or fish supplies 7 grams of protein, which corresponds to 7,000 milligrams of amino acids! Thus, dietary sources of protein such as chicken or beans are in fact a "time release" source of amino acids.

Endurance athletes have also been encouraged by advertisements in popular athletic magazines to consume specific amino acids during exercise to improve endurance, and again following exercise to enhance their recovery. Branched-chain amino acids—leucine, isoleucine, and valine—are broken down for energy during prolonged endurance exercise. These amino acids are important nitrogen sources for the amino acid alanine, which is converted to glucose to help fuel endurance exercise. However, obtaining adequate quantities of branched-chain amino acids from food is easy, and because they don't improve performance, endurance athletes don't require supplements.

Problems with High-Protein Diets and Supplements

Athletes who eat sufficient calories and get 12% to 15% of their calories from protein don't need protein supplements. The average diet already provides ample protein for muscle growth and repair. There is no evidence that protein supplements enhance muscle development, strength, or endurance. Extra protein doesn't help and may hurt health and performance.

Your body can't tell the difference between protein obtained from food and from expensive protein supplements. Many athletes don't realize that when they eat more protein than they require, the excess protein is either burned for energy or converted to fat. Burning protein for energy is expensive and wasteful. Carbohydrates are a more effective and less costly source of energy.

Consuming too much protein, whether from food or supplements, increases the body's water requirement and may contribute to dehydration. This occurs because the kidneys need more water to eliminate the excessive nitrogen load imposed by a high-protein intake. Athletes on high-protein diets should be sure to drink additional fluids to avoid becoming dehydrated.

High-protein diets are also usually high in fat. Consuming a high-protein, high-fat diet after heavy training will cause incomplete replacement of muscle glycogen and so impair performance. Digesting this type of diet also takes a long time, and such a diet can contribute to feelings of sluggishness. By comparison, a high-carbohydrate diet is easily digested and quickly restores muscle glycogen. High-fat diets can also increase the risk of health problems. Athletes on a high-protein diet should emphasize protein sources that are low in fat (nonfat dry milk powder, tuna in water, and beans).

Athletes who are determined to take protein supplements can use nonfat dry milk powder. It is a high-quality, inexpensive protein supplement (1/4 cup provides 11 grams of protein) without the unproven additives such as chromium and amino acids that many protein or "weight gainer" supplements contain.

There may be unidentified long-term risks associated with amino acid supplementation. Large intakes of some amino acids may interfere with the absorption of certain essential amino acids. When the body's proportion of amino acids is unbalanced, or if an essential amino acid is missing, the body can actually lose protein.

Taking ornithine supplements can cause mild to severe stomach cramping and diarrhea. Other amino acids alter nerve transmission in the brain. Some, such as methionine, are very toxic. Last, substituting amino acid supplements for food may cause deficiencies of other nutrients found in protein-rich foods, such as iron, niacin, and thiamin.

There is no evidence that supplementation with specific amino acids will improve endurance, increase muscle mass, or decrease body fat. It makes no sense to consume a product that has not been proven safe or effective, particularly when that product is promoted by people who stand to gain financially by its sale.

8

Vitamins and Minerals

Is More Better?

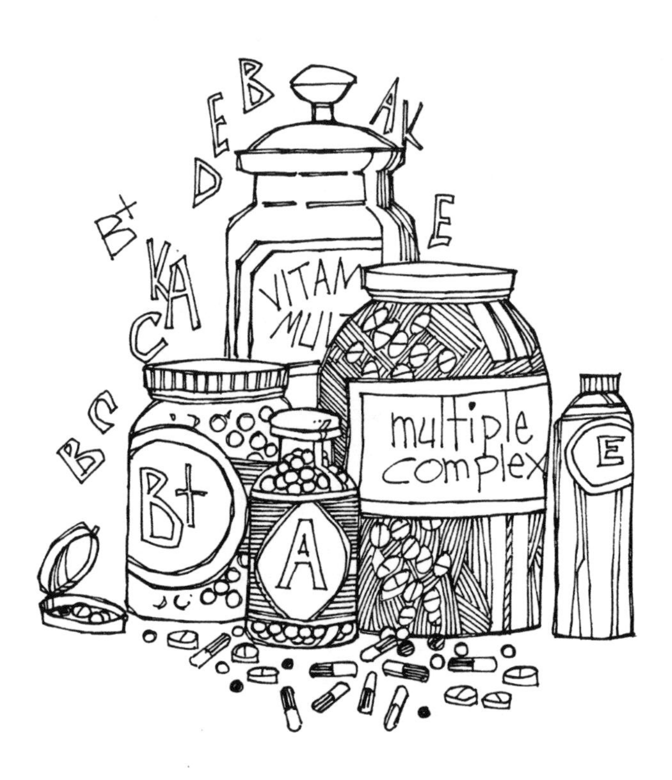

I was working with an athlete who was taking loads of vitamins.

"Is it okay to take all these vitamins?" he asked me.

I told him about the possible hazards of taking high doses, then asked: "Do you notice any difference?"

The only thing he'd noticed was that his urine was very yellow.

"What about your performance? Are you doing any better?" I asked him.

"I hope so," he said. "I've spent so much money on vitamins that I'd like to think they're doing something."

NUMEROUS ADVERTISEMENTS claim that athletes and active people require large doses or special mixtures of vitamins and minerals to support their active lifestyles. Many people assume that if a small amount of nutrient is good, more will be better. In addition to seeking a competitive edge, athletes may feel that their diets are inadequate and take supplements for "nutritional insurance." Athletes generally don't need or benefit from vitamin/mineral supplements. However, two minerals —calcium and iron—are of special concern for female athletes.

Vitamins

Vitamins are organic molecules that the body cannot manufacture but requires in small amounts. They are metabolic regulators that help govern the processes of energy production, growth, maintenance, and repair. Thirteen vitamins have been identified; each has a specific function in the body and also works in complicated ways with other nutrients.

In small amounts, vitamins function as catalysts—substances that increase the speed of a reaction without being used up by the reaction. This explains why they are needed in only small amounts (see Table 8-1).

Contrary to popular belief, vitamins do not provide energy, although some vitamins are important for the

TABLE 8-1
U.S. RECOMMENDED DIETARY ALLOWANCES (RDA) FOR VITAMINS

ADULT U.S. RDA FEMALE/MALE	FUNCTIONS	SOURCES
Vitamin C 60 mg	Aids collagen formation; enhances immunity; is antioxidant	Citrus fruits, tomatoes, strawberries, potatoes, broccoli, cabbage
Vitamin B_1 *(Thiamine)* 1.1/1.5 mg	Aids energy production and central nervous system maintenance	Meat, whole-grain cereals, milk, beans
Niacin 15/19 mg	Aids energy production and synthesis of fat and amino acids	Peanut butter, whole-grain cereals, greens, meat, poultry, fish
Vitamin B_6 *(Pyridoxine)* 1.6/2.0 mg	Helps protein metabolism, hemoglobin synthesis, and energy production	Whole-grain cereals, bananas, meat, spinach, cabbage, lima beans
Folacin 180/200 mcg	Aids new cell growth and red blood cell production	Greens, mushrooms, liver
Vitamin B_{12} *(Cobalamin)* 2 mcg	Aids energy metabolism, red blood cell production, and central nervous system maintenance	Animal foods
Vitamin A 800/1,000 mcg	Protects vision, skin; is antioxidant; enhances immunity	Milk, egg yolk, liver, yogurt, carrots, greens
Vitamin D 5 mcg	Helps formation of bones; aids absorption of calcium	Sunlight, fortified dairy products, eggs, fish
Vitamin E 8/10 mg	Is antioxidant; protects unsaturated fats in cells from damage	Vegetable oils, margarines, grains
Vitamin K 65/80 mcg	Aids blood clotting	Greens, liver

release of energy from food. Only protein, carbohydrate, and fat provide energy (calories). Consequently, the vitamin requirements of an active person are generally not greater than those of a sedentary person.

Thiamin, riboflavin, and niacin are exceptions because they are required in proportion to calories consumed, and active people need more calories. However, a balanced diet provides ample amounts of these vitamins. They are supplied by those carbohydrate-rich foods recommended for athletes—bread and whole-grain or enriched-grain products.

Vitamins are divided into two groups—water soluble and fat soluble. Fat-soluble vitamins include A, D, E, and K. They are not excreted but instead are stored in body fat, principally in the liver. Taking a greater amount of vitamins A and D than the body needs over a period of time can produce serious toxic effects.

Vitamins C and the B complex are soluble in water and must be replaced on a regular basis. When you consume more water-soluble vitamins than you need, the excess is eliminated in the urine. Though this increases the vitamin content of your urine, it doesn't help your performance. Consuming excessive amounts of water-soluble vitamins, such as niacin and B_6, can also cause dangerous side effects.

Recommended Dietary Allowances

The National Academy of Sciences has established and regularly updates recommended dietary allowances (RDAs) as a guide for determining nutritional needs. The RDA is an amount of an essential nutrient that is scientifically judged to be adequate to meet the known nutrient needs of practically all healthy people.

The RDA is not the smallest amount required to prevent disease symptoms because it includes a large margin of safety. For example, the body requires about 10 milligrams of vitamin C daily to prevent the deficiency disease scurvy, but the RDA is set at 60 milligrams.

Many athletes feel that taking vitamin/mineral supplements is justified because the RDAs don't account for the varying nutritional needs of different people. In general, the nutrient needs for the average person are only about two-thirds of the RDA. This means that as long as athletes consume at least 67% of the RDA for a given nutrient, they are probably protected from a nutritional deficiency.

The RDA for vitamins also varies only slightly for people of different ages, sizes, and sexes. Generally, a large active man doesn't require significantly more vitamins than a small sedentary woman.

Minerals

Minerals are inorganic compounds that serve a variety of functions in the body (see Table 8-2). Some minerals, such as calcium and phosphorus, are used to build bones and teeth. Others are important components of hormones, such as iodine in thyroxin. Iron is crucial in the formation of hemoglobin—the oxygen carrier within red blood cells.

Minerals also contribute to a number of the body's regulatory functions. These include regulation of muscle contraction, conduction of nerve impulses, clotting of blood, and regulation of normal heart rhythm.

TABLE 8-2
U.S. RECOMMENDED DIETARY ALLOWANCES (RDA) FOR MINERALS

ADULT U.S. RDA FEMALE/MALE	FUNCTIONS	SOURCES
Calcium 800 mg	Bone formation, enzyme reactions, muscle contractions	Dairy products, green leafy vegetables, beans
Iron 15/10 mg	Hemoglobin formation, muscle growth and function, energy production	Lean meat, beans, dried fruit, some green leafy vegetables
Magnesium 280/350 mg	Energy production, muscle relaxation, nerve conduction	Grains, nuts, meats, beans
Sodium EMR* 500 mg	Nerve impulses, muscle action, body fluid balance	Table salt, small amounts in most food except fruit
Potassium EMR* 2,000 mg	Fluid balance, muscle action, glycogen and protein synthesis	Bananas, orange juice, fruits, vegetables
Zinc 12/15 mg	Tissue growth and healing, immunity, gonadal development	Meat, shellfish, oysters, grains
Copper ESI* 1.5/3 mg	Hemoglobin formation, energy production, immunity	Whole grains, beans, nuts, dried fruit, shellfish

TABLE 8-2
(CONTINUED)

ADULT U.S. RDA FEMALE/MALE	FUNCTIONS	SOURCES
Selenium 55/70 mcg	Antioxidant function, protection against free radicals, enhancement of vitamin E	Meat, seafood, grains
Chromium ESI* 50/ 200 mcg	Part of glucose tolerance factor—aid to insulin	Whole grains, meat, cheese, beer
Manganese ESI* 2/5 mg	Bone and tissue development, fat synthesis	Nuts, grains, beans, tea, fruits, vegetables
Iodine 150 mg	Metabolism regulation	Iodized salt, seafood
Fluoride 1.5/4 mg	Formation of bones and tooth enamel	Tap water, tea, coffee, rice, spinach, lettuce
Phosphorus 800 mg	Formation of bones and teeth, metabolism regulation	Meat, fish, dairy products, carbonated drinks

*EMR—estimated minimum requirement
*ESI—estimated safe and adequate dietary intake

Minerals are classified into two groups based on the body's need. Major minerals, such as calcium, are needed in amounts greater than 100 milligrams per day. For minor minerals or trace elements, such as iron, fewer than 100 milligrams per day are required. Calcium and iron are both minerals of concern for athletes, especially women.

Calcium and Osteoporosis

Calcium is the most abundant mineral in the body. The bones and teeth contain 99% of the body's calcium; the remaining 1% circulates in the bloodstream. Calcium is critical for conducting nerve impulses, for heart function, for muscle contraction, and for the operation of certain enzymes. When the supply of calcium in the blood is too low, the body withdraws calcium from the bones.

Osteoporosis is an age-related disorder in which bone mass decreases and the susceptibility to fractures increases. It is a major public health problem in our country. Osteoporosis is called the silent disease because it usually goes undetected until a fracture occurs, often in the hip, wrist, or spine. Dual photon absorptiometry is an accurate way to measure bone mineral mass with minimal radiation exposure.

Estrogen loss and inadequate calcium intake contribute to osteoporosis. Women are more susceptible to osteoporosis than men because of their lower bone mass and menopause-related decline in estrogen. Weight-bearing exercise and weight training enhance skeletal calcium absorption and increase the strength of the bone, thus exerting a protective effect against osteoporosis.

The RDA for calcium for adolescents and young adults up to age 24 is 1,200 milligrams per day. For adult men and women age 25 and above, the RDA is 800 milligrams per day. However, the National Institutes of Health (NIH) recommends that premenopausal adult women consume 1,000 milligrams per day. Women of any age who are on estrogen replacement therapy should also consume 1,000 milligrams per day as they can still lose bone mass. Postmenopausal women who are not on estrogen should consume 1,500 milligrams per day. Half of all adult women consume less than 500 milligrams of calcium per day.

Obtaining Adequate Calcium

Dairy products represent the best sources of calcium (see Table 8-3). An eight-ounce glass of milk or 1/3 cup of nonfat powdered milk contains about 300 milligrams of calcium. Skim or low-fat versions of milk, yogurt, cottage cheese, or cheese provide the same amount of calcium as the regular versions of these foods, but contain less fat and calories.

Other good sources of calcium are sardines (because of the bones) and oysters. Broccoli and greens (kale, collard, turnip, and mustard) are good sources of calcium without any fat. Tofu that has been processed with calcium sulfate can also be a good source of calcium.

Many factors determine how much calcium is absorbed by the body. For example, high intakes of protein, sodium, and caffeine interfere with calcium retention by increasing the amount of calcium excreted in the urine. Excess alcohol intake also has detrimental effects on bone mass.

Before opting for a supplement, consult a registered

TABLE 8-3
SOURCES OF CALCIUM

MILK AND DAIRY PRODUCTS	MG
Milk, nonfat	300
Low-fat fruit-flavored yogurt	345
Low-fat plain yogurt	415
*Cottage cheese, 2%	138
*Cheddar cheese, 1 oz.	204
*Mozzarella, part skim, 1 oz.	183
*Parmesan, 1 oz.	390
Ricotta, part skim, 1 oz.	77
*Swiss, 1 oz.	272
Tofu, 3 1/2 oz.	127
FISH	**MG**
*Salmon, canned, 3 oz.	167
*Sardines, canned, 3 oz.	326
WATER	**MG**
"Hard" water, 1 qt.	100
"Soft" water, 1 qt.	30
NUTS, LEGUMES	**MG**
Almonds, 1/2 cup	173
Lentils, cooked	50
Dried beans, cooked	90
VEGETABLES	**MG**
Certain leafy green vegetables, including dandelion greens, mustard greens, turnip greens, collards, and kale, *but* excluding spinach, beet greens, and chard	280

All quantities are 1 cup unless indicated otherwise. Some good sources of calcium are also high in sodium, indicated with an asterisk (*). If you are not restricting sodium too much, you can still include these in your diet.

SOURCE: Nash, Joyce D. (1997). *Maximize your body potential,* 2nd ed. Palo Alto, CA: Bull Publishing. Used with permission.

dietitian or physician for advice on how to obtain the appropriate amounts from food and supplements. Too much calcium can be detrimental. In some people, excessive calcium intake increases the risk of urinary tract stones. Therefore, calcium intake should not exceed recommended levels.

Calcium carbonate (Tums® or a generic equivalent) is an inexpensive and acceptable calcium source. Calcium carbonate is 40% calcium, so a 500 milligram tablet actually provides 200 milligrams of elemental calcium. Such antacids that contain calcium are practically the same as dietary supplements. The primary difference between the two is in the marketing—when calcium carbonate is marketed as a calcium supplement, it costs more.

Bone meal and dolomite should not be used as calcium supplements because they may contain harmful amounts of lead, arsenic, mercury, and other potentially toxic minerals.

Athletic Amenorrhea

Some women who exercise strenuously stop menstruating, a condition called athletic amenorrhea. It is associated with low body weight/low body fat, nutritional inadequacy, physical stress and energy drain, and acute and chronic hormonal alterations. Although the specific cause of athletic amenorrhea is unknown and may vary among women, it appears to coincide with decreased estrogen production. When the athlete participates in a sport emphasizing leanness, however, the amenorrhea may be the result of disordered eating (see Chapter 15).

In the early 1990s, a strong relationship was recognized between disordered eating (anorexia), menstrual dysfunction (amenorrhea), and bone mineral disorders (reduced bone mineral density and increased risk of fractures). These have been termed the athletic female triad. Because estrogen deficiency is an important risk factor for the development of osteoporosis, athletic amenorrhea may increase the female athlete's risk of stress fractures and early osteoporosis.

Spinal bone mass has been found to be lower in amenorrheic women runners than in normal women runners. Further follow-up of these women indicated that bone mineral density remained well below the average for their age group 4 years after the resumption of normal menstruation.

Amenorrheic women athletes are not advised to stop exercising. In fact, exercise may partially overcome the calcium withdrawal from the skeleton associated with estrogen deficiency. Women who have athletic amenorrhea should consult a physician to rule out any serious medical problems, and all amenorrheic women should consume 1,500 milligrams of calcium daily. Regardless of menstrual function, most female athletes need to increase their calcium intake to meet the RDA for calcium.

After consultation with a physician, several strategies may be recommended to promote the resumption of menstruation. These include estrogen replacement therapy, weight gain, diet modification, and reduced training.

Iron

Iron deserves special attention because of the prevalence of iron-deficiency anemia—the nation's most common nutritional deficiency. Iron is needed to form hemoglobin, an iron-containing protein that carries oxygen in the blood and releases it to the tissues. When the total hemoglobin concentration drops, the muscles do not receive as much oxygen.

Hemoglobin levels below 12 grams per deciliter (gm/dl) for women and below 14 gm/dl for men are considered diagnostic for anemia. Anemic people have less endurance and cannot exercise as strenuously as people who are not anemic. Their aerobic capacity is reduced because of the decreased oxygen-carrying capacity of their blood.

Women, compared to men, are much more likely to suffer from iron-deficiency anemia. Iron deficiency in women is usually the result of menstrual blood loss and inadequate dietary iron intake. There is also evidence that strenuous training accelerates the destruction of red blood cells, possibly from mechanical trauma (such as hitting the ground with the feet while running) and gastrointestinal bleeding. Exercise increases the iron lost in sweat and may decrease iron absorption from the gut.

Male and female endurance athletes must take special care to consume the RDA for iron—10 milligrams for men and 15 milligrams for women. Women athletes typically consume only 10 milligrams per day.

Obtaining Adequate Iron

Animal sources of iron should be emphasized, as the iron from them is better absorbed than the iron from vegetable sources. Combining animal and vegetable products (such as a meat and bean burrito) increases the iron absorbed from the vegetable product. Vitamin C also enhances iron absorption, so high vitamin C foods (e.g., orange juice) should be consumed with foods containing iron (e.g., iron-fortified cereals) for optimum absorption.

Cast-iron cookware can increase the iron content of foods. The more acidic (e.g., spaghetti sauce) and the longer the food is cooked in cast-iron cookware, the higher will be the residual iron content of the food.

Red meat is an excellent iron source, containing about 1 milligram of iron per ounce. Iron-enriched or fortified cereal/grain products can contribute significantly to the iron content of the diet. Beans, peas, split peas, and some dark green leafy vegetables are also good vegetable sources of iron (see Table 8-4).

Despite the prevalence of anemia and the difficulty of obtaining enough iron, female athletes shouldn't routinely take iron supplements. That tired, listless feeling can be caused by numerous conditions. Self-supplementation of iron (even at RDA levels) can be particularly dangerous.

Women at risk for iron deficiency should have their hemoglobin levels checked periodically. A more sensitive but expensive test for iron deficiency also measures serum ferritin. Low ferritin levels appear in the first stage of iron deficiency, representing inadequate iron stores in your bone marrow. This test is valuable because it detects iron deficiency early, before iron-deficiency anemia develops. A low ferritin level can mean that the person has an increased risk for developing iron-deficiency anemia. Knowing that iron levels are low allows an individual to increase her iron stores through a greater intake of iron to head off the consequences of anemia.

Iron supplementation will not improve the health or performance of a woman with normal iron stores. On the

TABLE 8-4
SOURCES OF IRON

FOOD	MEASURING UNIT	IRON (MG)
*Liver—pork	3 oz.	17.7
*Liver—lamb	3 oz.	12.6
*Liver—chicken	3 oz.	8.4
*Liver—beef	3 oz.	6.6
*Oysters, fried	3 oz.	5.9
Tostada, bean	1	3.2
Dried apricots	1/2 cup (12 halves)	3.0
Baked beans with pork and molasses	1/2 cup	3.0
Soybeans, cooked	1/2 cup	2.7
*Beef	3 oz.	2.7
*Beef enchilada	1	2.6
Raisins	1/2 cup	2.5
Lima beans, canned or fresh cooked	1/2 cup	2.5
Refried beans	1/2 cup	2.3
Dried figs	1/2 cup (4 figs)	2.2
Spinach, cooked	1/2 cup	2.0
*Taco—beef	1	2.0
Mustard greens, cooked	1/2 cup	1.8
Corn tortilla, lime treated	8 inch diameter	1.6
Prune juice	1/2 cup	1.5
Peas, fresh cooked	1/2 cup	1.4
Enchilada, cheese and sour cream	1	1.4
Egg	1 large	1.2
*Turkey, roasted	3 oz.	1.1
Sardines, canned in oil	1 oz. (2 medium)	1.0

*Foods of animal origin. Iron in foods of animal origin (except milk, which has little iron) is absorbed twice as efficiently as iron in foods of plant origin.

SOURCE: Smith, Nathan J., & Worthington-Roberts, Bonnie. (1989). *Food for sport.* Palo Alto, CA: Bull Publishing. Used with permission.

other hand, excessive intake can produce an iron overload (especially if a person absorbs too much iron) and cause deficiencies of the trace minerals copper and zinc. Iron supplements should not exceed the RDA unless medically indicated and prescribed by a physician.

Supplementation Concerns

High doses of vitamins (amounts 10 times the RDA for water-soluble vitamins; 5 times the RDA for fat-soluble vitamins) can be dangerous. When vitamins are taken in such huge amounts, they no longer function as vitamins; they become drugs and may produce serious side effects.

Vitamins A and D in particular can build up in the body to toxic levels. Too much vitamin A can cause neurological problems, including brain damage. Too much vitamin D can cause destructive deposits of excess calcium in soft tissues like the kidneys and lungs.

Large doses of water-soluble vitamins can also cause side effects. Large amounts of niacin can cause severe flushing, liver damage, ulcers, and blood sugar disorders. High doses of niacin also interfere with fat metabolism and speed up glycogen depletion.

Excess vitamin B_6 (pyridoxine) has caused neurological symptoms similar to multiple sclerosis in women who have taken supplements to alleviate premenstrual symptoms. Large doses of vitamin C can cause diarrhea, kidney stone formation, and impaired copper absorption.

Like fat-soluble vitamins, excess amounts of minerals are also stored in the body and can build up to toxic levels.

An excess of one mineral can interfere with the functioning of others. Because iron overload can damage the liver, pancreas, and heart, iron supplements should be used only for proven iron deficiency. Although about 6% of Americans are iron deficient and will benefit from iron supplementation, more than 10% of Americans have excess iron in their bodies and can be harmed by iron supplements.

Supplement Recommendations

Does anyone need vitamin/mineral supplements? The Council on Scientific Affairs of the American Medical Association (AMA) has published a report on the appropriate use of supplements. Healthy adult men and women who aren't pregnant or breast-feeding do not require supplements—provided that they're eating a balanced and varied diet.

The council concedes that changing dietary habits (increased consumption of processed and fast foods) may cause instances in which vitamin intake is inadequate. Before opting for supplementation, however, people should try to improve their food selection and eating habits.

The Committee on Diet and Health (Food and Nutrition Board, National Research Council) recommends that people avoid taking dietary supplements that exceed 100% of the RDA in any one day. Most people can, and should, obtain essential nutrients from a variety of foods.

The committee noted possible exceptions: women who are pregnant or breast-feeding, women with excess monthly bleeding, people on very low calorie diets, some vegetarians, and people with malabsorption problems. However, these individuals should be evaluated on a case-by-case basis before taking supplements.

The AMA Council condemns the increasing use of megadose therapy because it is based on testimonial, non-scientific evidence. Megadose therapy only thins wallets and builds false hopes, without providing any beneficial results. More important, the consumption of large amounts of vitamins and minerals can produce toxic effects and/or upset the delicate balance of these nutrients.

Most health authorities agree that there is no harm in a simple vitamin/mineral supplement, provided it does not exceed 100% of the RDA for nutrients. Keep in mind there is also no evidence that this supplementation is beneficial.

Supplements and Athletes

Supplementation at levels exceeding the RDA does not improve the performance of well-nourished athletes. Although vitamin and mineral deficiencies can impair athletic performance, active people rarely have such deficiencies. There is a close relationship between caloric intake and vitamin intake: The more food a person eats, the greater will be the vitamin intake. Athletes generally eat more than sedentary people and so tend to get more vitamins and minerals in relation to their needs.

Athletes who limit their caloric intake are at risk for nutritional deficiencies. These athletes usually compete in sports that emphasize leanness for enhanced performance (runners, wrestlers, lightweight crew) or for appearance (gymnasts, figure skaters, divers, ballet dancers). Weight-conscious active people may also be at risk. A vitamin/mineral supplement supplying no more than 100% of the RDA might be appropriate for some of these individuals.

Athletes often feel that their run-down feeling is due to a vitamin or mineral deficiency. When there is a nutritional reason for fatigue, it is usually an inadequate intake of calories or carbohydrate. Athletes who are always tired may be eating too little carbohydrate or calories for glycogen synthesis, or they may be overtraining. When athletes feel better after taking vitamin/mineral supplements, it's probably because of the power of their belief that supplements help—the placebo effect.

Nutrients and Peak Performance

No one food or food group supplies all the nutrients you need, so you should choose a wide variety of foods from the five groups in the pyramid. Eat at least the minimum number of servings from each food group daily to get the nutrients you need for peak performance.

Of the 40 known nutrients, 10 are considered leader nutrients. If you obtain adequate amounts of these nutrients from the foods you eat, you will probably obtain the other 30 nutrients as well. The 10 leader nutrients are protein, carbohydrate, fat, vitamin A, vitamin C, thiamin, riboflavin, niacin, calcium, and iron.

The five food groups in the Food Guide Pyramid were developed based on these leader nutrients. The foods in the grain group are high in carbohydrate, thiamin, niacin, and iron. The fruit and vegetable groups contain foods high in vitamins A and C. Meat group foods are high in protein, niacin, iron, and thiamin. Foods in the milk group are good sources of calcium, riboflavin, and protein.

Taking vitamin/mineral supplements is easier than changing eating habits. Supplements provide the illusion that you are caring for your health, but they remove the burden of dietary change. You can't improve performance just by taking a pill. Supplements don't improve a balanced diet or "fix" a deficient diet. For nutritional insurance, you should eat more complex carbohydrates and fewer empty calories (sugar, fat, and alcohol).

9

Hydration

Don't Forget to Drink

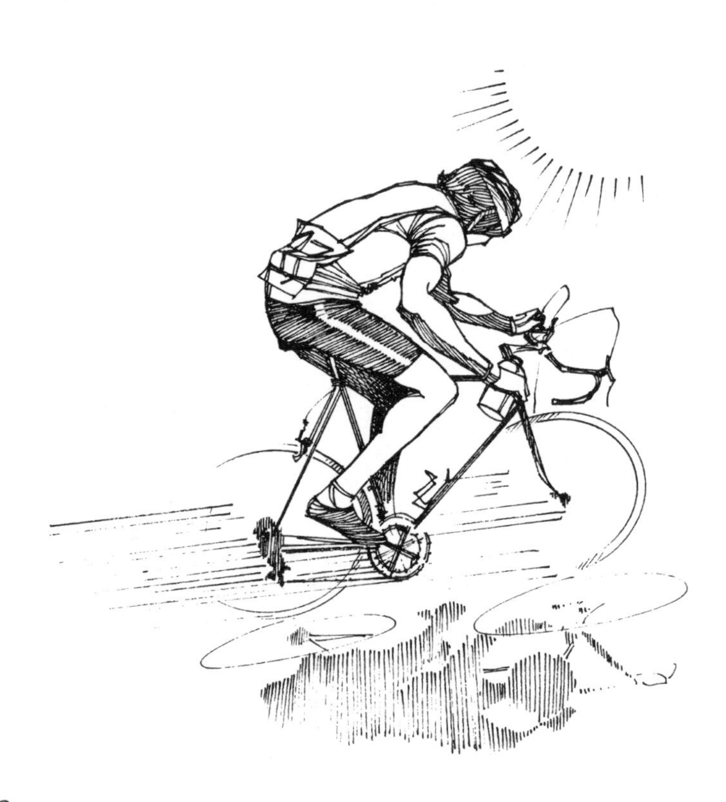

I was the second person to get to the lunch stop at the 100-mile mark of a 200-mile ride. The temperature was 100 degrees F., and I was tired.

I started the second 100 miles with two full water bottles. No shade. Hilly steep pitches. I was going very slowly and still felt terrible, riding in my lowest gear. Ten miles out I had gone through both water bottles.

There was no escape from the heat. Cycling produced more heat. Raging thirst. I searched for water but the hills were parched. I felt they would find my bleached bones on the side of the road.

I became disoriented and was on the verge of crying. Not thinking clearly, I went on for 30 more miles. Rounding a corner I thought I saw a bicyclist in need of help and stopped. There was no one there. I was hallucinating.

Other experienced riders felt the same thing—throbbing heads, hot/cold flashes, and sudden weakness. Only 20% of those who started the race finished. The environment was so harsh that we couldn't drink enough fluids to replace our losses.

Water is the most important of all nutrients, as your body requires it constantly. An adequate supply of water is essential for temperature control (particularly during exercise), for energy production, and for elimination of waste products from metabolism. Dehydration—the loss of body water—reduces endurance and increases the risk of heat illnesses (heat exhaustion and heat stroke). Water is probably the nutrient most neglected by athletes.

Water and Temperature Regulation

Considering the dollars spent on supplements in pursuit of a competitive edge, it is amazing how often athletes ignore the importance of fluids. Consuming cool fluids at regular intervals during exercise is vital for safeguarding health and optimizing athletic performance.

Water acts as a coolant to keep the body from overheating during physical activity. During exercise, heat is generated as a by-product of the working muscles. When heat builds up, the body temperature rises. This heat must be removed to maintain a normal body temperature.

During exercise in warm weather, sweat is the body's main mechanism for getting rid of excess heat. When sweat evaporates from the skin, the body cools down. Large sweat losses, however, harm athletic performance and hinder the body's ability to control body temperature. The reason is that during exercise in the heat, blood that was transferring oxygen to the muscles is diverted to skin to help eliminate heat. The competition for blood between the muscles and skin places a greater demand on your cardiovascular system. At the same time, your blood volume is decreasing because of sweat losses. As you become dehydrated, both your heart rate and your body temperature increase.

Your body is programmed to protect its cardiovascular function at the expense of body temperature regulation. Consequently, skin blood flow and sweat rate are decreased in an effort to conserve body fluid. As a result, your body temperature rises and you experience fatigue and increased risk of heat injury (see Figure 9-1).

In practical terms, when you're dehydrated you can't exercise as hard or as long. During prolonged exercise in the heat, sweat losses constituting as little as 2% of your body weight impair athletic performance and temperature regulation. Athletes can dehydrate by 2% to 6% of their body weight despite the availability of fluids. Inadequate fluid replacement speeds up dehydration and can ultimately cause a life-threatening heat illness.

You may be unaware of the huge sweat losses that can occur during hot, dry weather. Large amounts of fluid evaporate very quickly in these conditions. Because you don't feel sweaty, you may not realize how much water you've lost.

Besides heat, relative humidity is also important. As the moisture in the air increases, the effectiveness of evaporation through sweating decreases. If the air is saturated with water, little evaporation will occur even at cooler temperatures and body heat can build up. When sweat drips off your skin, you're not getting the cooling benefit of sweat.

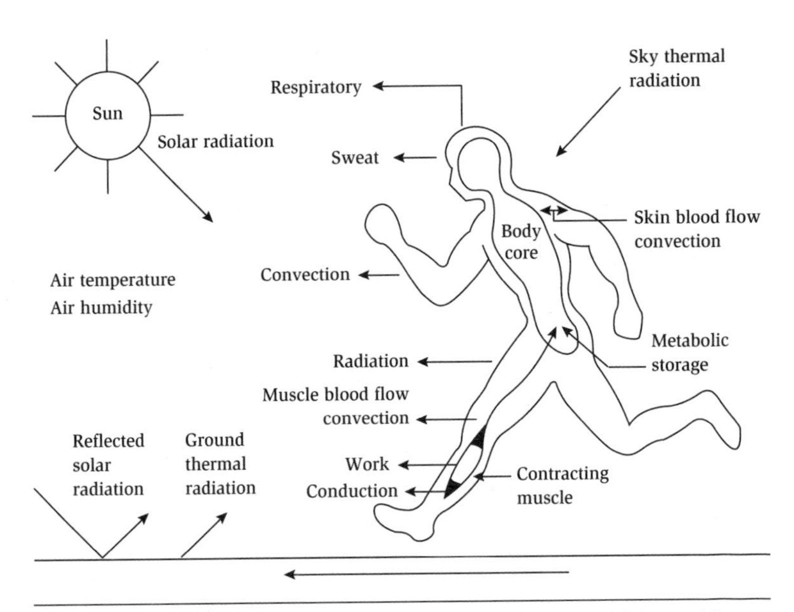

FIGURE 9-1. Schematic diagram showing heat production within working skeletal muscle, its transport to the body core and to the skin, and its subsequent exchange with the environment.

SOURCE: Reprinted with permission of Macmillan Publishing Company from *Exercise and Sport Scientist Reviews,* Vol. 12, by V. C. Gisolfi, C. G. Wenger. Copyright 1984 by American College of Sports Medicine.

Be aware of intense physical exertion on warm, humid days as well as on hot, dry days.

If you wear a sweat suit, there is no opportunity for evaporation. People who exercise in sweat suits (or worse, full rubber suits during hot weather) to lose weight or get in shape endanger their health and even their lives. Any extra weight loss is just water, which will be replaced.

Be aware of the symptoms of impending heat illness. These include weakness, feeling of chills, goose pimples on the chest and upper arms, nausea, headache, faintness, disorientation, muscle cramping, and cessation of sweating.

If you continue to exercise when you experience any of these symptoms, you can sustain a heat injury.

Heat Illnesses

Athletes who exercise in hot or humid weather are at risk for heat cramps, heat exhaustion, or heat stroke. Three factors contribute to the development of heat injuries: increased body temperature, loss of body fluids, and loss of electrolytes.

Heat cramps

Heat cramps, or involuntary muscle spasms, occur during or after activity, usually in the specific muscles exercised. Heat cramps are probably caused by an imbalance of the body's fluid and electrolyte concentrations. Muscle spasms can occur if the electrolytes lost in sweat aren't replaced. The treatment is to rest, drink fluids with electrolytes such as sport drinks, and add salt to foods.

Heat exhaustion

Heat exhaustion is probably caused by a reduced blood volume resulting from excessive sweating. Blood then pools in the extremities and the person may faint or feel dizzy. The symptoms of heat exhaustion also include nausea and fatigue. Although sweating may be reduced, the rectal temperature is not elevated to dangerous levels (less than 104 degrees F.). The treatment is to rest in a cool place and drink fluids containing electrolytes. Medical attention may be required.

Heat stroke

Heat stroke is a medical emergency requiring immediate action. The body's temperature-regulating processes simply stop functioning. Sweating usually stops and the skin becomes dry and hot. The rectal temperature is excessively high—over 105.8 degrees F. Other symptoms include disorientation, vomiting, headache, and unconsciousness. If untreated, the condition leads to death that occurs due to circulatory collapse and central nervous system damage. The treatment requires that aggressive steps be taken immediately to lower the elevated body temperature. Until medical help arrives, cover the person with ice packs, immerse him in cold water, or rub him with alcohol.

Fluid Replacement Guidelines

At rest, you need at least two quarts of fluid daily. Exercise greatly increases your fluid requirements. You can prepare for exercise in the heat by drinking 16 ounces of rapidly absorbed fluid (water or sports drink) two hours before exercise. This technique is called hyperhydration; it helps to lower your body's core temperature and reduce the added stress that heat places on your cardiovascular system.

Drinking during exercise is essential to prevent the detrimental effects of dehydration on your body temperature and exercise performance. You should drink 5 to 10 ounces of rapidly absorbed fluid every 15 to 20 minutes during exercise. Obviously, the actual amount you consume will vary based on your rate of dehydration from sweating.

There is no safe level of dehydration that you can tolerate before cardiovascular function and temperature regulation are impaired (see Table 9-1). You'll perform at your best when your fluid intake closely matches your fluid losses from sweating.

Thirst is not an adequate guide to fluid replacement. Most people replace only 50% of their fluid losses during

TABLE 9-1
ADVERSE EFFECTS OF DEHYDRATION

% BODY WEIGHT LOSS	SYMPTOMS
0.5	Thirst
2.0	Stronger thirst, vague discomfort, loss of appetite
3.0	Increasing hemoconcentration, dry mouth, reduction in urine
4.0	Increased effort for exercise, flushed skin, impatience, apathy
5.0	Difficulty in concentrating
6.0	Impairment in exercise temperature regulation, increased heart rate
8.0	Dizziness, labored breathing in exercise, mental confusion
10.0	Spastic muscles, inability to balance with eyes closed, general incapacity, delirium and wakefulness, swollen tongue
11.0	Circulatory insufficiency, marked hemoconcentration and decreased blood volume, failing renal function

SOURCE: Greenleaf, J. E., & Fink, W. J. (1982). Fluid intake and athletic performance. In W. Haskell (Ed.), *Nutrition and athletic performance.* Palo Alto, CA: Bull Publishing. Used with permission.

exercise. You need to regulate your fluid intake by drinking according to a time schedule rather than in response to thirst.

Get in the habit of regular drinking during training. Some athletes pay attention to their fluid intake only during competition and become dehydrated in workouts. Heat injury can occur just as easily during training. Adequate fluid intake during training protects against heat illness and enables you to get the most out of your workouts. It also gives you the chance to practice proper hydration techniques.

Weigh yourself before and after exercise (nude is best) to determine how much fluid you're losing. Drink 16 ounces of fluid for every pound of body weight lost. If you notice a gradual loss of weight during warm weather training, you may be experiencing chronic dehydration rather than body fat loss. Urine that is dark in color may also indicate a dehydrated state.

Fluid Replacement Beverages

You can consume water or a sports drink to replace fluid losses (see Table 9-2). Sports drinks containing carbohydrate and sodium such as Gatorade are absorbed as quickly as water. The presence of glucose and sodium in sports drinks increases fluid uptake in the small intestine.

Sports drinks promote optimum cardiovascular function and temperature regulation as well as plain water. However, unlike water, sports drinks improve performance during prolonged exercise by providing carbohydrate for the working muscles. For exercise lasting an hour or longer, sports drinks provide a performance edge that water can't. Sports drinks are also beneficial when you're exercising for an hour several times a day. However, water remains an effective and inexpensive fluid replacement beverage for exercise lasting less than an hour.

For optimal absorption and performance, a sports drink should contain 6% to 8% carbohydrate—about 60 to 80 calories per 8 ounces. It is doubtful that drinks containing less than 5% carbohydrate—about 50 calories per 8 ounces—will help performance. Those that exceed 10% carbohydrate, about 100 calories per 8 ounces—fruit juices, sodas, and concentrated fructose drinks—take longer to be absorbed and can cause abdominal cramps, nausea, bloating, and diarrhea.

Fluid replacement beverages should be rapidly absorbed, taste good, and not cause gastrointestinal problems when consumed in large volumes. Beyond these concerns, it's a matter of personal preference. Try several different sports drinks during training to find the one that works the best for you.

Electrolytes

Electrolytes such as sodium, chloride, and potassium are necessary for the maintenance of body fluid levels, muscle contraction, and nerve impulse transmission.

Sweating causes electrolyte losses (particularly sodium) as well as water losses. However, water losses during sweating are proportionately greater than electrolyte losses, so the body's cells actually end up with a greater electrolyte concentration.

TABLE 9-2
FLUID REPLACEMENT BEVERAGES

BEVERAGE	FLAVORS	CARBO-HYDRATE INGREDIENT
Gatorade® Thirst Quencher The Gatorade Company	Lemon-lime, orange, fruit punch, lemonade, citrus cooler, tropical fruit, grape, iced tea cooler	Powder: sucrose and glucose; Liquid: Sucrose and glucose/ syrup solids
Powerade® Coca Cola	Lemon-lime, fruit punch, orange, grape	High fructose corn syrup, maltodextrin
AllSport® Pepsico	Lemon-lime, fruit punch, orange, grape	High fructose corn syrup
10-K® Suntory Water Group, Inc.	Lemon-lime, orange, fruit punch, lemonade, iced tea, pink lemonade, apple	Sucrose, glucose, fructose
Quickick® Quick Kick	Lemon-lime, orange, fruit punch	High fructose corn syrup
Endura® Meta Genics, Inc.	Orange, lemon-lime	Glucose polymers, fructose
1st Ade® American Beverages	Lemon-lime, orange, fruit punch	High fructose corn syrup fructose
Hydra Fuel® Twin Labs	Orange, fruit punch, lemon-lime	Glucose polymers, glucose, fructose
Cytomax® Champion Nutrition	Fresh apple, tropical fruit, cool citrus	Corn starch, fructose, glucose
Gookinaid® Gookinaid ERG	Lemon, fruit punch orange	Glucose
Pro Motion® Sports Beverage	Lemon-lime, fruit punch, orange citrus cooler	Fructose

Table 9-2
(continued)

Carbohydrate % (Concentration) Per 8 Oz.	Sodium (Mg) Per 8 Oz.	Potassium (Mg)	Other Minerals and Vitamins
6	110	30	Chloride, phosphorus
8	55 or less	30	Chloride
8	55	55	Chloride, phosphorus, calcium
6	55	30	Vitamin C, chloride, phosphorus
7	100	23	Calcium, chloride, phosphorus
6	46	80	Calcium, chloride, magnesium, chromium
7	55	25	Phosphorus
7	25	50	Chloride, magnesium, chromium, phosphorus, vitamin C
5	53	100	Chromium, magnesium
12	70	70	Vitamins A and C, calcium, iron
7.7	8	99	None

(continued)

TABLE 9-2
(CONTINUED)

BEVERAGE	FLAVORS	CARBO-HYDRATE INGREDIENT
Everlast Sports Drink® A & W Beverages, Inc.	Lemon-lime, orange, mixed berry, grape	Sucrose, fructose
PurePower® Energy & Recovery Drink Purepower Sports Nutrition	Lemon-lime, apple, tropical fruit	Fructose, maltodextrin
Breakthrough® Weider Health & Fitness	Lemon, tangerine, fruit punch, grape	Maltodextrin, fructose
Coca-Cola®	Regular, cherry	High fructose corn syrup, sucrose
Diet soft drinks	All	None
Orange juice	—	Fructose, sucrose
Water	0	0

**TABLE 9-2
(CONTINUED)**

CARBOHYDRATE % (CONCENTRATION) PER 8 OZ.	SODIUM (MG) PER 8 OZ.	POTASSIUM (MG)	OTHER MINERALS AND VITAMINS6 100
6	100	20	Vitamin C
4.3	50	100	Chromium, vitamin C, calcium, phosphorus, magnesium
8.5	60	45	Vitamin C, calcium, chloride, magnesium, riboflavin, niacin, iron, thiamin
11	6	Trace	Phosphorus
0	2–8	18–100	Low phosphorus
10	6	436	Vitamins A and C, niacin, thiamin, riboflavin
0	Low	Low	Low

Your electrolyte needs can generally be met by consuming a balanced diet. Although sodium is the major electrolyte lost in sweat, our diets provide an abundance of salt (sodium chloride). The loss of one gram of sodium, which occurs with a two-pound sweat loss, can easily be replaced by moderate salting of food. One-half teaspoon of salt supplies one gram of sodium.

Salt tablets should be avoided entirely. They can cause nausea by irritating the stomach lining and increase your body's water requirement.

Replacing potassium losses should not be a problem either. You lose far more sodium than potassium during exercise. Orange juice, bananas, and potatoes are all excellent sources of potassium. Potassium supplements are unnecessary and can be dangerous. They can cause an excessively high level of potassium in the blood, resulting in an abnormal heart rhythm.

Electrolyte deficits, particularly sodium, can occur under certain conditions—when you are acclimating to a hot environment, following repeated workouts in hot weather, and during ultra-endurance events such as 50-mile runs, 100-mile bicycle rides, and long triathlons (such as the Ironman).

Consuming only plain water during ultra-endurance events can cause a dangerous condition called hyponatremia (low blood sodium). Sodium losses in sweat during ultra-endurance events can be significant, and when you drink only water, you dilute the amount of sodium left in the blood.

Symptoms of low blood sodium include lethargy, muscle cramping, mental confusion, and seizures. Fortunately, this condition is rare; heat illnesses occur far more often.

Hyponatremia can be prevented by consuming sports drinks that contain sodium.

Because sports drinks contain less sodium than found in sweat, consuming them can't cause a sodium overload. In addition to aiding fluid absorption during exercise, the sodium in sports drinks encourages fluid intake because it makes the drink taste better.

Sports drinks containing sodium can promote rehydration after exercise. The sodium helps to maintain your thirst and keeps you drinking while it delays urine production. This combination promotes rapid rehydration and enhances your recovery. Drinking plain water eliminates your thirst so that you stop drinking, and urine production is stimulated. This sequence delays rehydration and can hinder your recovery.

Alcohol

Drinking too much alcohol before endurance exercise (even the night before) can harm performance. Alcohol is a diuretic; it causes increased urination and water loss. The dehydrating effect of alcohol impairs performance and increases the risk of heat illnesses during exercise in warm weather.

Alcohol is a central nervous system depressant that reduces gross motor skills such as balance and coordination. It is metabolized by the liver, which can get rid of only about a half-ounce of alcohol per hour. Drinking alcohol before or during exercise decreases the output of glucose by the liver, thereby causing low blood glucose levels and early fatigue. Consuming alcohol during exercise in cold weather may also contribute to hypothermia (dangerously low body temperature).

Alcohol is a concentrated source of calories but does not contribute to the formation of muscle glycogen, the primary fuel for exercise. One 12-ounce beer or 5-ounce glass of wine supplies only 50 calories of carbohydrate—enough to run a half mile. At the same time, these drinks supply one-half ounce of pure alcohol—a detrimental chemical responsible for traffic accidents and health problems.

Twelve ounces of beer, 5 ounces of wine, and 1 1/2 ounces of hard liquor contain about equal quantities of alcohol. One or two drinks of this size daily appear to cause no harm to nonpregnant, healthy adult athletes who can afford the calories. Pregnant women should not drink, as consumption of alcohol may cause birth defects or other problems during pregnancy.

Alcoholic beverages are high in calories and low in nutrients—a source of empty calories for adult athletes who wish to reduce their body fat. Athletes who drink should substitute alcohol calories for fat calories—not food calories. One 12-ounce beer provides 150 calories. Five ounces of wine or 1 1/2 ounces of liquor each supplies about 100 calories.

10

The Sugar Debate

Poison or Pleasure?

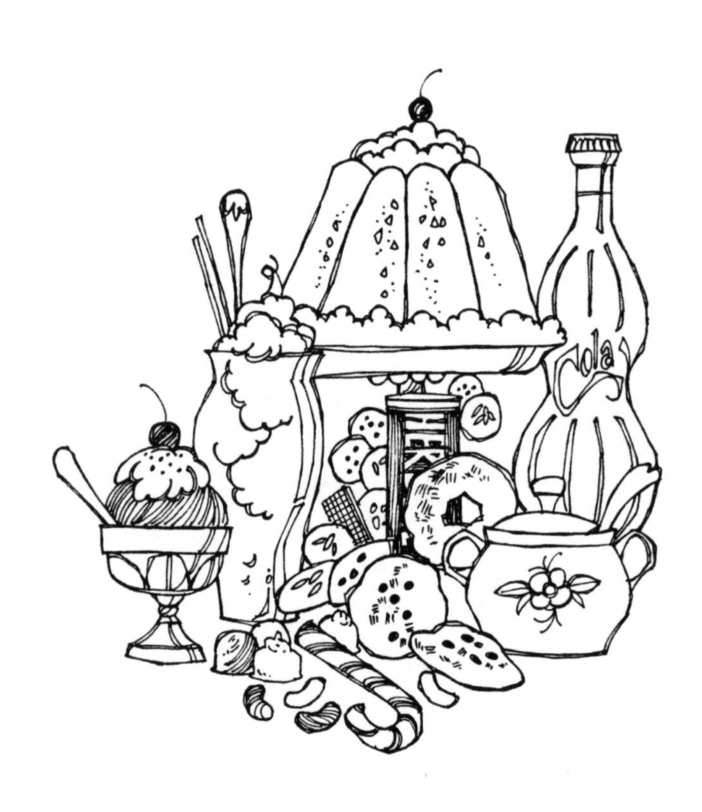

I was trying to finish the 200-mile ride in less than 11 hours. At the 130-mile mark, though, I weakened. I knew I needed food and accepted some glucose tablets from another rider. I probably ate 300 calories of straight glucose all at once.

Zap! Fifteen miles later I experienced severe gut cramps. For the last 50 miles the gas pains became so terrible I thought I would have to stop.

I must have had an awful fluid imbalance in my intestines. Though I achieved my goal, I would have felt much better if I had spaced those tablets out.

SUGAR IS NOT A POISON. When eaten appropriately, it can be very helpful to the athlete. There are simple rules for how much to eat, when to eat it, and in what form. Some athletes eat large quantities of sugar (and/or honey) in the belief that it is a high-energy food and will improve endurance or speed. Others try to avoid it entirely, believing that sugar is detrimental to athletic performance and health. The better position is somewhere between these extremes.

Carbohydrate Before Exercise

Athletes are often warned not to eat large amounts of sugar or starch prior to exercise. This advice was based on research conducted in the late 1970s, which suggested that consuming 75 grams of glucose (300 calories) 30 minutes prior to exercise reduced endurance by causing hypoglycemia (low blood sugar) and early fatigue. The impaired performance was thought to occur due to high blood insulin levels induced by the pre-exercise sugar feeding.

Insulin is secreted by the pancreas in response to an increase in blood glucose. Insulin promotes the uptake of glucose into cells and lowers the blood glucose level. When the blood glucose drops too low, the person may experience hypoglycemic symptoms (weakness, dizziness, nausea, confusion, and partial blackout) or become exhausted sooner.

Fortunately, these insulin and glucose responses are temporary and probably will not harm performance. In fact, research conducted since 1989 shows that consuming carbohydrate (sugar or starch) before exercise may help your performance. Consuming carbohydrate prior to exercise lasting an hour or longer provides glucose for your muscles to use when they're running low on glycogen. More on this when we discuss the pre-event meal in Chapter 12.

The results of both the old and new studies suggest that people differ in sensitivity to having their blood glucose lowered. Most people won't be affected by a temporary drop in blood glucose, but a few may feel weak and tired. The physiological basis for this difference is unknown.

Be aware that consuming sugar an hour prior to exercise may harm your performance if you're sensitive to having your blood glucose lowered. You can test yourself in training to see whether you develop any symptoms or become exhausted sooner. However, the only real way to find out is to have your blood glucose level measured.

If you think you are sensitive to pre-exercise sugar or starch feedings, consume your carbohydrate either a few minutes before exercise or wait until you're exercising. The rise in the exercise hormones (epinephrine and growth hormone) blocks the release of insulin and in that way counters insulin's effect in lowering blood glucose.

Carbohydrate During Exercise

Carbohydrate feedings during endurance exercise lasting an hour or longer may enhance endurance by providing glucose for muscles to use when their glycogen stores have dropped to low levels. Consuming carbohydrate while you are exercising at 70% of your $\dot{V}O_{2max}$ can delay fatigue for 30 to 60 minutes.

The liver supplies glucose to maintain blood glucose for proper functioning of the central nervous system. As the muscles run out of glycogen, they will begin to take up some of the blood glucose, placing a drain on the liver glycogen stores. The longer the exercise session, the greater will be the utilization of blood glucose by the muscles for energy.

When the liver glycogen is depleted, the blood glucose level drops. Though a few athletes experience symptoms indicative of hypoglycemia, most athletes are forced to reduce their exercise intensity because of muscle fatigue.

The improved performance associated with carbohydrate feedings during exercise results from the maintenance of blood glucose levels. Dietary carbohydrate supplies glucose for the muscles at a time when their glycogen stores are diminished. Thus, the production of ATP from carbohydrate can continue at a high rate and endurance is enhanced. Remember: ATP (energy) production is faster from carbohydrate than from fat.

Endurance athletes should consume 30 to 60 grams of carbohydrate (120 to 240 calories) every hour. You can obtain this amount from either carbohydrate-rich foods (sports bars, fruit, grain products, liquid meals) or sports drinks (see Chapter 12). Sports drinks are a practical source of carbohydrate because they replace fluid losses as well.

Try to eat before you feel tired or hungry, usually within 30 minutes into exercise. Consuming small amounts at frequent intervals (every 30 to 60 minutes) will help prevent gastrointestinal upset. Your foods and fluids should be easily digestible, familiar (tested in training), and enjoyable (to encourage eating and drinking).

Sugar During Training

Sugary foods such as cakes, cookies, pies, soft drinks, and candy can be helpful for increasing carbohydrate and calorie intake during training. However, these foods should be eaten in addition to, and not in place of, complex carbohydrate foods. When sugar replaces complex carbohydrates in the diet, your intake of vitamins, minerals, and fiber will be reduced. Remember that sugar can also contribute to tooth decay. Many sugary baked goods and candy are also high in fat.

Sugar Myths

Despite popular press claims, brown sugar, date sugar, honey, and molasses are not nutritionally superior to table sugar. Though these so-called natural sugars do contain trace amounts of some vitamins and minerals, consuming them will not add significant nutritional value to your diet.

Some endurance athletes take fructose, thinking it is superior to glucose or other sugars. Fructose causes a lower insulin response than glucose, a quality that has led some athletes to think it is a better energy source.

However, consuming fructose does not improve endurance and has even been shown to harm performance. You store twice as much muscle glycogen after eating glucose or sucrose than you do after eating fructose.

Also, fructose is far more likely to cause gastrointestinal distress, even in small amounts. For this reason, glucose, maltodextrins (glucose polymers), and sucrose are the major carbohydrate sources in sports drinks. Maltodextrins are created by breaking down corn starch into small glucose chains (polymers).

Consuming sugar before anaerobic exercise such as sprinting or weight lifting will not improve performance because the body relies on stored ATP and muscle glycogen for these tasks. It won't provide you with a sudden burst of energy, allowing you to exercise harder or longer. To the contrary, eating too much sugar immediately before or during exercise can increase the risk of gastrointestinal problems in the form of cramps, nausea, diarrhea, and bloating.

The Role of Complex Carbohydrates and Fruit

Your primary carbohydrate source should be the grain products, beans, vegetables, and fruit found at the bottom of the Food Guide Pyramid (Figure 4-1). These foods promote good health and athletic performance. Grain products, beans, vegetables, and fruit supply vitamins, minerals, and fiber along with their carbohydrate.

The dietary fiber found in whole grains, vegetables, and fruit may reduce your risk of heart disease and certain cancers. The soluble fiber found in beans, fruit, oats, and vegetables can help lower the cholesterol level in your blood. Because high blood cholesterol is a major risk factor for heart disease, consuming more soluble fiber may help reduce your risk for heart disease. Fruits and vegetables high in beta-carotene and vitamin C may also help to prevent some kinds of cancer.

Insoluble fiber found in whole-grain products and bran speeds up the movement of food through the gastrointestinal tract. It may reduce your risk for colon cancer and other bowel disorders. Insoluble fiber also provides a feeling of satiety, which is important for weight control and can alleviate constipation.

Grain products, fruits, and vegetables are nutrient dense—they supply a significant amount of nutrients for their calories. Compare a small baked potato with a third of a candy bar, both of which contain about 100 calories. The potato provides ample vitamin C, a small amount of protein, B vitamins, about half a dozen minerals, and fiber. The third of the candy bar provides the same amount of energy, about three times as much fat, and little or no fiber, vitamins, and minerals.

Contrary to popular belief, starches such as bread, cereal, potatoes, corn, beans, rice, and pasta contribute significantly fewer calories for a given amount than foods with a high fat or sugar content. The "diet lunch" of a hamburger patty and a scoop of cottage cheese provides a lot of fat calories.

By replacing fats and sugary foods in the diet, complex carbohydrates actually facilitate weight loss because they contain fewer calories. Also, the naturally occurring sugars in fruit make them ideal for a sweet, low-calorie treat.

11

Caffeine

Unraveling the Caffeine Controversy

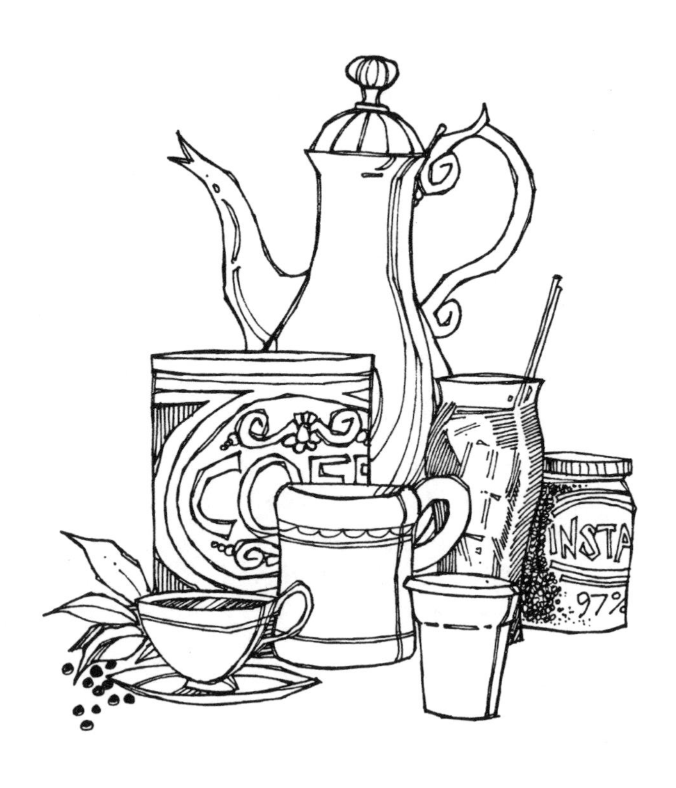

When the initial findings about the effects of caffeine were published, the man who presented the research was touted as a caffeine-pusher. Those people who didn't drink coffee took issue with his findings.

Those people who had enjoyed coffee for years were elated that something good had been found in what they considered to be a bad habit.

Actually, he was an honest researcher who simply wanted to publish his findings without bias.

Caffeine can improve endurance in dosages below the International Olympic Committee (IOC) doping threshold. However, it doesn't work for everyone and there is an ethical question regarding the use of caffeine to improve performance. Caffeine holds a unique position in the athletic world. The use of caffeine is restricted by the (IOC) in that urinary caffeine levels above 12 micrograms per milliliter are considered illegal. However, caffeine is an integral part of many athletes' diets, and moderate caffeine doses (3–6 milligrams per kilogram of body weight) can enhance endurance performance. Thus, caffeine has the potential to be a legal and safe performance aid.

Caffeine and Endurance

The interest in caffeine as an endurance aid was initiated by research published between 1978 and 1980. In a 1978 study, cyclists who consumed 330 milligrams of caffeine (5 milligrams per kilogram of body weight) 1 hour prior to cycling at 80% of $\dot{V}O_{2max}$ were able to ride 19% longer (90 minutes compared to 75 minutes) prior to reaching exhaustion. A 1979 study showed that consuming 250 milligrams of caffeine was associated with a 20% increase in the amount of work that could be performed in 2 hours.

These two studies suggested that the utilization of fat for energy increased by about 30% in the caffeine trials. A third study in 1980 found that consuming 5 milligrams of caffeine per kilogram of body weight reduced muscle glycogen usage by 42% and increased muscle triglyceride usage by 150% during 30 minutes of cycling at 70% of $\dot{V}O_{2max}$.

Following these studies, good research on caffeine and performance was limited, and the results were inconsistent. However, since 1990 an impressive body of research has established that caffeine can improve endurance performance.

In a 1991 study, competitive distance runners were given 9 milligrams of caffeine per kilogram of body weight 1 hour prior to cycling and running to exhaustion at intensities of about 85% of $\dot{V}O_{2max}$. The average increase in endurance for the running test was 44%; for the cycling test, it was 51%. However, the urinary caffeine levels in one-third of the caffeine trials resulted in levels near or above the IOC threshold.

A review of caffeine research indicates that consuming 3 milligrams to 13 milligrams of caffeine per kilogram of body weight can improve the endurance performance by 20% to 50% in elite and recreationally trained athletes who run or cycle at 80% to 90% of their $\dot{V}O_{2max}$. In fact, a dose of only 3 milligrams to 6 milligrams of caffeine per kilogram of body weight improves performance without raising urinary caffeine levels above the IOC doping threshold.

Although higher doses also improve performance, about one-fourth of athletes who consume 9 milligrams of caffeine per kilogram of body weight will exceed the IOC limit, and two-thirds of those who consume 13 milligrams of caffeine per kilogram of body weight will exceed the IOC limit. Side effects of caffeine consumption (dizziness, headache, insomnia, and gastrointestinal distress) are also more common at doses of 9 milligrams to 13 milligrams per kilogram of body weight, but they are infrequent with doses at or below 6 milligrams per kilogram of body weight.

How does caffeine enhance endurance? Because caffeine affects both the central nervous system and skeletal muscles, separating out its effects is not possible. Conceivably, different mechanisms are responsible for performance improvement in different exercise situations.

Three major theories have been proposed for the performance-enhancing effects of caffeine. First, as a well-known central nervous system stimulant, caffeine increases a person's alertness and decreases the sensation of fatigue. Caffeine may reduce the perception of effort by lowering the threshold for nerve transmission and muscle fiber recruitment, making it easier to recruit the muscles for exercise.

Second, caffeine may increase the force of muscle contractions by improving sodium-potassium pump activity and calcium movement within the exercising muscles.

Third, caffeine may increase fat utilization and decrease carbohydrate utilization. This is the metabolic hypothesis that was proposed by caffeine researchers in the late 1970s. Caffeine may mobilize free fatty acids from adipose or intramuscular triglyceride by increasing circulating epinephrine levels. The increased availability of free fatty acids increases fat metabolism and decreases carbohydrate utilization. This delays glycogen depletion and so enhances endurance performance.

Caffeine does produce a twofold increase in plasma epinephrine (at rest and during exercise) and a twofold increase in plasma free fatty acids at rest. However, the elevation in free fatty acids lasts for only the first 15 to 20 minutes of exercise. Muscle glycogen usage is reduced following caffeine consumption, but this glycogen sparing effect is limited to the initial 15 minutes of exercise at 80% of $\dot{V}O_{2max}$. Although these metabolic effects partly explain how caffeine improves endurance, the other theories cannot be ruled out.

If you want to try caffeine, experiment with it in training first. The dose recommended to improve endurance is between 3 milligrams and 6 milligrams per kilogram of body weight, taken one hour before exercise (see Table 11-1). Side effects of high caffeine consumption include nausea, muscle tremors, palpitations, and headache. Some people are extremely sensitive to caffeine and ingesting it won't improve their performance. Athletes who are sensitive to caffeine can experience these symptoms at low doses.

What about the well-known diuretic effect of caffeine? In theory, caffeine could cause you to become dehydrated and increase your risk of heat illness. The good news is that none of the studies evaluating caffeine's metabolic and performance effects suggest that caffeine increases the risk of heat illness. If you drink properly before, during, and after exercise, the suggested caffeine dose shouldn't be a problem.

However, you may want to avoid caffeinated beverages after exercise when you are trying to replace your fluid losses. A study examined the effectiveness of rehydrating

TABLE 11-1
SOURCES OF CAFFEINE

COFFEE (5-OZ. CUP)			
Espresso	150 mg	Instant	40–108 mg
Drip	110–150 mg	Decaffeinated (instant)	2 mg
Percolator	64–124 mg	Decaffeinated (brewed)	2–5 mg
SOFT DRINKS (12 OUNCES)			
Diet Mr. Pibb	59 mg	Sunkist Orange	42 mg
Mountain Dew	54 mg	Dr. Pepper	40 mg
Tab	47 mg	Sugar-free Dr. Pepper	40 mg
Coca-Cola, Diet Coke	46 mg	Pepsi	38 mg
Shasta Cola, Diet Cola	44 mg	Diet Pepsi, Pepsi Light	36 mg
Shasta Cherry Cola	44 mg	Royal Crown Cola	36 mg
Shasta Diet Cherry Cola	44 mg	Diet Rite	36 mg
TEA (5-OZ. CUP)			
Black tea brewed 5 min	20–50 mg	Green tea	30 mg
Black tea brewed 3 min	20–46 mg	Instant tea	12–28 mg
Black tea brewed 1 min	9–33 mg	Ice tea (12-oz. can)	22–36 mg
DRUGS (PER TABLET)			
Pain Relievers		Diet/Weight Control	
Excedrin	64–130 mg	Dexatrim	200 mg
Anacin, Emprin, or Vanquish	32 mg	Dietac	200 mg
Aspirin (plain)	0 mg	Prolamine	140 mg
Feminine Needs		Alertness/Stimulants	
Pre Mens Forte	100 mg	Vivarin	200 mg
Pre Mens	66 mg	NoDoz	100–200 mg
Midol	32–65 mg		
Diuretic			
Aqua-Ban	200 mg		
Permathene	200 mg		

Note: Products change from time to time, and caffeine content may also change.

SOURCE: Adapted from Nash, Joyce D. (1997). *The New Maximize Your Body Potential*, 2 ed. Palo Alto, CA: Bull Publishing. Used with permission.

after exercise with diet caffeinated soda, a sports drink containing 6% carbohydrate, and water. Compared to the sports drink and water, the diet caffeinated soda (frequently chosen by weight-conscious athletes) was poor at replacing fluid losses because it increased the production of urine.

The Ethical Issue

Although caffeine provides performance benefits when urinary levels are well below the IOC's limit, serious ethical issues are raised regarding the use of caffeine to improve performance. Even when caffeine is used in legal amounts, it may be considered a form of doping, thereby violating the ethics of sports performance. The American College of Sports Medicine, the United States Olympic Committee, and the American Dietetic Association do not endorse the use of caffeine to enhance endurance.

12

Eating for Performance

The High-Performance Diet

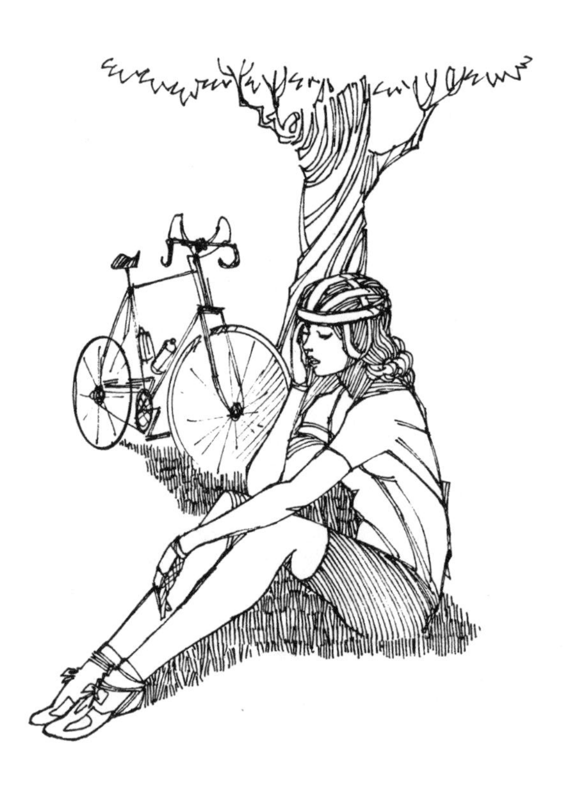

After 10 grueling hours—four in 90-degree heat, we had reached the last rest stop, the 170-mile mark of a 200-mile cycling race. I was sunburned, breathing hard, hurting. Lying on the ground I ate about five chocolate chip cookies, wondering if I could ride another 30 miles. My chief adversary rode up and my heart sank—she looked great. We had been riding neck and neck and she seemed definitely to be the stronger one. I knew she hadn't taken a rest or eaten since the 150-mile mark. "C'mon," she said to a friend. "Let's go pick up my trophy."

I dragged myself back onto my bike and gave chase. It was sheer determination and concentration on my part that kept my legs moving. My competitor was talking and making jokes, looking like she was part of her cycle. About 10 miles later she began to fade as I perked up.

"What's the matter?" I asked her.

"I don't know," she said. "I feel weak and shaky."

Slowly the roles reversed. I felt strong. She faded off the back of the pace line. I pulled the pace line into the finish for the last 15 miles—finishing strongly and feeling great.

Later, I learned that my competitor had stopped about 10 miles out. She ordered a shake at a fast food restaurant and fainted. It had been almost 3 hours since she had eaten.

THERE IS A GREAT DEAL OF CONFUSION about what to eat before, during, and after training and competition. To some degree it is an individual matter. Only you can truly learn what works for you—by trial and error well before competition. The length of your event also makes a difference; there are guidelines for events of varying duration.

Pre-Exercise Eating

Athletes often train or compete in the morning without eating. This overnight fast lowers your liver glycogen stores (the source of blood glucose) and can impair performance during prolonged endurance exercise that relies heavily on blood glucose.

During exercise, you rely primarily on your pre-existing muscle glycogen and fat stores. Although the pre-exercise meal doesn't contribute immediate energy for exercise, it can provide energy when you exercise for longer than an hour. It can also prevent you from feeling hungry, and hunger in itself may impair performance.

Athletes are often advised to eat 2 to 3 hours prior to exercise to allow adequate time for stomach emptying. The rationale is that if any food remains in the stomach when you start exercising, you can become nauseated when blood is diverted from the stomach to the exercising muscles. Rather than getting up at the crack of dawn to eat, many athletes who exercise in the morning simply forego eating.

Athletes have also been instructed to avoid high-carbohydrate foods immediately before exercising. The concern is that carbohydrate may elevate blood insulin at the start of exercise, resulting in hypoglycemia and fatigue during the exercise. As discussed in Chapter 10, eating carbohydrate before exercise will probably help, not hurt, your performance.

Eating a high-carbohydrate meal before morning exercise can help restore liver glycogen stores, and these replenished levels will help you during prolonged exercise. If muscle glycogen levels are also low, the meal can help to increase them as well if you eat several hours before exercise.

Consume 1 to 4 grams of carbohydrate per kilogram of body weight, 1 to 4 hours before exercise. To avoid potential gastrointestinal distress, reduce the size of the meal—making it smaller as it is consumed closer to exercise time. For example, a carbohydrate feeding of 1 gram per kilogram of body weight (4 calories per kilogram) is appropriate an hour before exercise, whereas 4 grams per kilogram (16 calories per kilogram) can be consumed 4 hours before exercise.

Good examples of high-carbohydrate foods for pre-exercise meals include fruit, bread products (adding jam or jelly increases the carbohydrate content), and nonfat or low-fat yogurt. Fruit juices and nonfat milk are good high-carbohydrate beverages. You can also use liquid meals or high-carbohydrate liquid supplements.

Fatty foods should be limited because they delay stomach emptying and can contribute to a heavy, sluggish feeling. Many high-protein foods eaten at breakfast (eggs, cheese) are also high in fat. In contrast, carbohydrates provide the quickest and most efficient source of energy and, unlike fats, are rapidly digested.

High-fiber foods should be limited as they may cause abdominal cramping and necessitate a bathroom break during exercise. This is merely annoying during training, but it can be disastrous during competition.

You should test the effectiveness of your pre-exercise meal in training, not before an important competition.

Liquid Meals

A number of commercially formulated liquid meals are also available (see Table 12-1). Their fluid and carbohydrate content make them a desirable meal choice.

Liquid meals have several advantages over conventional meals. They leave the stomach more rapidly than regular meals, which helps to avoid pre-competition nausea. Liquid meals also produce a low stool residue, which helps to keep immediate weight gain to a minimum. Because they don't contain fiber, liquid meals are also less likely to necessitate a bathroom break during exercise.

Liquid meals can also be used for nutritional supplementation during heavy training when caloric requirements are very high. They contribute a significant number of calories as well as a feeling of satiety. Liquid meals can also provide energy during prolonged exercise.

Homemade liquid meals can be concocted by mixing milk, fruit, and nonfat dry milk powder in a blender. For added variety, cereal, yogurt, and flavoring (vanilla and chocolate) can be added. Sugar or honey may also be added for additional sweetness and carbohydrate. Also, several brands of "instant breakfast" powders that can be mixed with milk are available.

TABLE 12-1
NUTRITION BEVERAGES

BEVERAGE	FLAVORS	CALORIES PER 8-OZ. SERVING	CARBOHYDRATE (GRAMS)	PROTEIN (GRAMS)	FAT (GRAMS)
GatorPro® Sports Nutrition Supplement The Gatorade Company	Chocolate, vanilla	360	58	16	7
Sport Shake® Mid-America Farms	Chocolate, vanilla, strawberry	310	45	11	10
Endura Optimizer® Unipro, Inc.	Chocolate, vanilla, orange	260	57	11	less than 1
Sego Very® Pet, Inc.	Chocolate, chocolate malt, strawberry, vanilla	180	27–34	9	1–4
Protein Repair Formula® PurePower Sports Nutrition	Vanilla	200	26	20	1.5
Metabolol II® Champion Nutrition	Plain	260	40	20	2
Ensure Ross Laboratories	Chocolate, strawberry, vanilla	254	35	9	9
Nutrament® Mead Johnson Nutritionals	Chocolate, banana, vanilla, strawberry, coconut	240	34	6.5	11
Sustacal® Mead Johnson Nutritionals	Chocolate, vanilla, strawberry, eggnog	240	33	5.5	14.5

Events Lasting 90 Minutes or Less

The recommended training diet for moderate training (6 to 8 grams of carbohydrate per kilogram of body weight, 1.2 grams to 1.4 grams protein and the remainder fat) provides adequate muscle glycogen stores for events lasting 90 minutes or less. You need to exercise longer than 90 minutes to benefit from carbohydrate loading.

A pre-event meal may improve your performance if you're exercising longer than an hour; follow the guidelines to avoid gastrointestinal problems. Consuming 3 to 6 milligrams of caffeine per kilogram of body weight an hour before the event (as discussed in Chapter 11) may allow you to exercise harder, particularly if you're exercising for an hour or more.

Proper hydration is your major nutritional concern during the event, as heat exhaustion and heat stroke can occur in runs as short as 6.2 miles. Drink 5 to 10 ounces every 15 to 20 minutes (as discussed in Chapter 9). Sports drinks may give you a performance boost if you're exercising an hour or longer.

Events Lasting 90 Minutes to 3 Hours

When you're training 2 hours or more per day, you should consume the amount of carbohydrate recommended for heavy training—8 grams to 10 grams per kilogram of body weight daily. This amount will help prevent training glycogen depletion, as discussed in Chapter 4. Protein should supply 1.2 grams to 1.4 grams per kilogram of body weight, and fat will provide your remaining calories.

You can carbohydrate load (as discussed in Chapter 5) to increase your muscle glycogen stores in the days prior to competition. Remember: Training too heavily the week prior to competition can predispose you to early muscle glycogen depletion. You can also consume 3 to 6 milligrams of caffeine per kilogram of body weight an hour before exercise to improve your endurance.

Eating a meal before the event will improve your endurance. In fact, consuming a high-carbohydrate pre-exercise meal adds to the benefit you get from consuming carbohydrate during exercise. During the event, your primary need is fluid. Drink 5 to 10 ounces every 15 to 20 minutes.

When you're exercising longer than 60 minutes, you should consume 30 to 60 grams of carbohydrate (120 to 240 calories) every hour to improve endurance (as discussed in Chapter 10). This amount can be obtained through carbohydrate-rich foods (sports bars, fruit, and grain products) or sports drinks. Start taking in carbohydrate early, within the first half-hour of exercise.

Each carbohydrate form (liquid or solid) has advantages and drawbacks. Sports drinks are a practical source of carbohydrate because they also replace your fluid losses. They provide the right proportion of water to carbohydrate to promote rapid fluid replacement and provide energy for peak performance.

However, high-carbohydrate foods can be easily carried and provide a feeling of satiety that you won't get from drinking fluids. Drink plenty of water when you eat solid foods such as sports bars. Otherwise, the food can settle poorly and you may feel there's a rock in your gut. In addition to aiding your digestion, drinking water while eating solid foods encourages you to hydrate adequately.

Drinking 5 to 10 ounces of a sports drink containing 6% to 8% carbohydrate (e.g., Gatorade and Exceed) every 15 to 20 minutes supplies the right amount of carbohydrate. Eating one banana, four graham crackers, four fig bars, or one sports bar (e.g., Power Bar, TigerSport Bar) every hour also provides the recommended amount of carbohydrate (see Table 12-2).

Three Hours and Beyond

When you are training 2 hours or more daily, eat the diet recommended for heavy training: 8 to 10 grams of carbohydrate per kilogram of body weight, 1.2 to 1.4 grams of protein per kilogram, and the remaining calories from fat. If you are training longer than 3 hours a day, you may benefit from a carbohydrate intake greater than 10 grams per kilogram. Cyclists often consume 13 grams of carbohydrate per kilogram of body weight daily in the grueling Tour de France.

You can carbohydrate load, ingest caffeine, and eat a high-carbohydrate meal before the event to improve your endurance. However, the improvement in performance with pre-exercise carbohydrate feedings is less than when smaller quantities of carbohydrate are consumed during exercise.

When you exercise for 3 hours or longer, the food and

TABLE 12-2
WHERE THE CARBS ARE
(BARS, BANANAS, AND A FEW OTHER FAVORITES)

	CALORIES	CARBOHYDRATES (GM)	PROTEIN (GM)	FAT (GM)
PowerBar	225	47	9	2
TigerSport Bar	230	40	11	3
PR Bar	200	23	13	6
Fig bars (4 small)	212	42	2	4
Grahams (4 crackers, 2 1/2 by 5 inches)	240	44	4	6
Bananas (1 1/2)	180	45	0	0

fluid you consume during the event is at least as important as what you have consumed in the days before the event. When you're exercising this long, you need to take in carbohydrate during exercise to provide glucose for the working muscles.

As outlined earlier, you can get carbohydrate from sports drinks and from high-carbohydrate foods—fruit, grain products, sports bars, and liquid meals. These foods should be easily digestible, familiar (what you are used to eating in training), and enjoyable (to encourage you to eat).

Try to limit foods high in fat and protein during the event because they are hard to digest. Such foods may cause competition for blood between your stomach and muscles; they may also cause nausea and vomiting.

Eat before you feel tired or hungry, within 30 minutes

into exercise. If you eat small amounts at frequent intervals (every 30 to 60 minutes), you'll be more likely to prevent gastrointestinal upsets.

Once again, proper hydration is the most important nutritional concern during prolonged exercise. You can have adequate muscle glycogen stores and blood glucose and still collapse from heat exhaustion or stroke. Consume fluids before you are thirsty, as early as 15 minutes into exercise, and continue drinking according to a set schedule, as discussed in Chapter 9. Table 12-3 suggests food and drinks that are appropriate for events of varying lengths.

Never try an untested food or fluid during competition. The result may be severe indigestion and/or impaired performance.

After Exercise

Replacing your muscle glycogen stores following strenuous training is important if you are to minimize chronic fatigue. Based on the time you spend training, you should consume 6 grams to 10 grams of carbohydrate per kilogram of body weight daily.

It is also important to consume carbohydrate immediately (within 30 minutes) after heavy exercise lasting several hours. A study compared glycogen storage when carbohydrate was consumed immediately after exercise to glycogen storage when carbohydrate consumption was delayed for 2 hours after exercise. When the carbohydrate feeding was delayed for 2 hours, glycogen storage was cut in half, as measured 4 hours after exercise.

TABLE 12-3
FOOD/FLUID FOR EVENTS OF VARYING LENGTHS

	LENGTH OF EVENT		
DIETARY INTAKE	0–90 MINUTES	1½–3 HOURS	3 HOURS AND UP
Pre-exercise meal 1–4 hours before exercise	May help beyond 60 minutes	May improve endurance	May improve endurance
Caffeine 1 hour before exercise	May help beyond 60 minutes	May improve endurance	May improve endurance
Sports drinks with 6% to 8% carbohydrate	May help beyond 60 minutes	May improve endurance	May improve endurance
Carbohydrate loading	May harm performance due to weight gain	May improve endurance	May improve endurance
High-carbohydrate foods/ "liquid meals" during exercise	Probably will not help	May improve endurance	May improve endurance

Consuming high-carbohydrate fluids and foods right after prolonged training and competitions increases your glycogen storage and may help you recover faster. Replacing muscle glycogen stores after exercise is particularly beneficial if you train hard several times a day as it will enable you to get the most out of your second workout.

Many athletes aren't hungry after heavy training. If you are not, consume a high-carbohydrate drink such as fruit juice or a commercial high-carbohydrate supplement. This will also promote rehydration.

Endurance athletes who exercise hard for several hours

a day should consume 1.5 grams of carbohydrate per kilogram of body weight within 30 minutes of exercise, followed by an additional feeding of 1.5 grams per kilogram of body weight 2 hours later. The first carbohydrate feeding could be a high-carbohydrate beverage and the second feeding could be a high-carbohydrate meal.

For example, a 70-kilogram man should take in 105 grams of carbohydrate within 30 minutes of exercise. This amount corresponds to 18 ounces of GatorLode. Two hours later, he could have two cups of spaghetti with a half cup of tomato sauce, which provides 70 grams of carbohydrate. Adding two pieces of French bread increases his carbohydrate intake to 100 grams.

The next nutritional strategy necessary for an adequate recovery is proper rehydration. It is essential that you fully rehydrate between workouts. Weigh yourself after exercising and drink 16 ounces of fluid for each pound lost (as discussed in Chapter 9). Consuming sports drinks following exercise can promote rehydration, thereby enhancing your recovery. The sodium in the sports drink enables you to retain water without inhibiting your thirst.

13

Body Composition

Debunking the Myth of Bathroom Scales

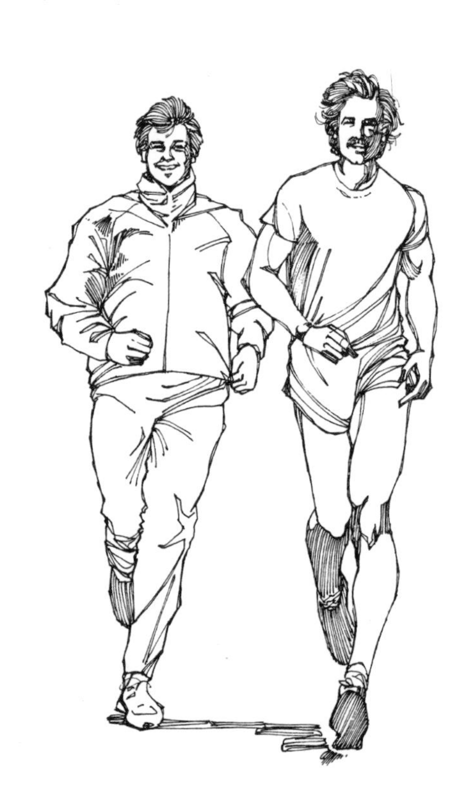

I worked with a muscular, well-built man about 5′7,″ 150 pounds, who decided that if he were thinner he could run better. He had looked at a height-weight table and decided he should weigh 135 pounds.

He cut his food intake, but kept his mileage the same. Not only did he have a difficult time losing weight, but his running form deteriorated. He lost his power and speed. He also became irritable, hungry, and began to fantasize about banana cream pie.

Before he tried to lose weight, I had evaluated his body composition and found that he had 7% body fat at 150 pounds. After his weight-loss attempt, I told him to throw his bathroom scale out the window and go back to his old diet. His running form soon returned to normal.

WE ARE A SOCIETY OBSESSED about weight. How many people do you know who talk constantly about "losing a few pounds"? What really counts is body composition: the amounts of fat-free mass and body fat. Athletes who want to maximize their potential should pay more attention to their body composition than their body weight.

The True Measure of Fatness

In our society, the bathroom scale has a following worthy of a political party or a religion. An unbelievable number of weight-loss gimmicks have been spawned by the American obsession about losing weight. Some of them endanger the health of their victims, others merely thin their wallets, and almost all fail to cause permanent weight loss. In the rush to shed pounds, a very important question is usually overlooked: "How fat am I?"

The scale cannot differentiate between fat pounds and muscle pounds. The scale does not indicate how fat a person is because both fat and muscle, as well as bone and water, contribute to the total weight.

The term *overweight* refers only to body weight in excess of the average weight for a specific height. The term *underweight* refers only to the body weight below the average weight for height. The scale is prejudiced against stocky, muscular people just as it is biased in favor of thin, slightly built people.

A more accurate indicator of fitness is body composition, which divides weight into two categories. One is fat-free mass, of which muscle is a major component. The other category is fat. What is really important is how much of a person's weight is fat. This is expressed as percentage of body fat.

People automatically assume that a gain in scale weight represents fat weight and that a loss in scale weight is fat loss. Thus, you often hear someone exclaim, "I've lost six pounds in one day!" It's physiologically impossible to lose six pounds of fat in one day. The person has actually lost water—which will be replaced. Fluctuations in scale weight do not necessarily represent changes in body fat, and that's what counts.

Body Shape and Size

Appearances can be very deceptive when it comes to estimating a person's percentage of body fat. When comparing the percentage of body fat of a marathon runner to that of a football player, most people would say that the marathon runner has less fat because he looks thinner. Yet, when evaluated, the football player may be as lean, in terms of percentage of body fat, as the runner.

Sure, the football player appears to be fatter, but this is because he is bigger. His weight and size are due to his enormous muscle mass. The runner, who in comparison may look like a prisoner of war, has proportionately less muscle mass. It is possible for two people to be 100 pounds apart in weight and have totally different body types, yet have the same percentage of body fat.

The person who suffers the most when evaluated by weight alone is the stocky, muscular man or woman. Though these athletes may have little fat, they weigh more than the average because of a large, fat-free mass. To lose weight, they may lose muscle and experience a deterioration in their performance. This is just one reason it is so important to have body composition assessed before trying to lose weight.

You are somewhat restricted by your genetic inheritance. Body shape and size are largely determined by skeleton size, as a certain amount of muscle and tissue accompany a certain amount of bone. Beyond heredity, your total amount and distribution of muscle mass will depend on the type of training you do. For example, weight training increases muscle mass more than distance running.

As athletes know, body type is important in most sports, and each sport seems to require a certain body type. The large, muscular person will never be an elite marathoner, just as the elite marathoner would not survive as an interior lineman on the football field.

Whereas body shape and size can be altered only slightly, substantial changes may occur in body composition. These changes can significantly affect your performance. In power sports, performance can be improved by the extra muscle gained from weight lifting. It is also obvious that performance in endurance sports can be harmed by excess body fat. However, an athlete who trains for a specific sport is likely to have the muscle mass that is appropriate for that sport. If, because of genetics, his muscle mass is greater than desired, he will only hurt himself by trying to starve himself thinner.

Body Composition

A healthy level of body fat for men is around 15%. A man is classified as obese when he exceeds 20% body fat. A healthy level of body fat for women is about 25%. A woman is classified as obese when she exceeds 30% body fat.

People who regularly participate in endurance exercise such as running, bicycling, and swimming usually have lower percentages of body fat, because the exercise both increases their lean body mass and uses up stored fat as fuel.

Three percent of the total body fat in men is considered essential fat. It appears that a man cannot reduce his body fat below this limit without impairing his physiological function and capacity for exercise.

The percentage of body fat considered essential for women is 12%. This higher level of fat is related to childbearing functions and takes into account sex-specific fat in the breasts and other tissues.

A number of studies have been done to assess the body composition of athletes. The results give body fat values that vary widely both between sports and within sports. Thus, an ideal percentage of body fat for a particular sport is difficult to establish. Table 13-1 shows percentage of body fat values for various types of athletes.

Before you attempt to achieve a certain percentage of body fat, you should be aware of several things. Your success in a sport depends on a variety of factors. Having a low percentage of body fat does not, in itself, ensure that you will be a good athlete.

TABLE 13-1
RANGES OF RELATIVE BODY FAT FOR MEN AND WOMEN ATHLETES IN VARIOUS SPORTS

SPORT	MEN	WOMEN
Baseball, softball	8–14	12–18
Basketball	6–12	10–16
Body building	5–8	6–12
Canoeing, kayaking	6–12	10–16
Cycling	5–11	8–15
Fencing	8–12	10–16
Football	6–18	—
Golf	10–16	12–20
Gymnastics	5–12	8–16
Horse racing	6–12	10–16
Ice and field hockey	8–16	12–18
Orienteering	5–12	8–16
Pentathlon	—	8–15
Racquetball	6–14	10–18
Rowing	6–14	8–16
Rugby	6–16	—
Skating	5–12	8–16
Skiing	7–15	10–18
Ski jumping	7–15	10–18
Soccer	6–14	10–18
Swimming	6–12	10–18
Synchronized swimming	—	10–18
Tennis	6–14	10–20
Track and field		
Running	5–12	8–15
Field events	8–18	12–20
Triathlon	5–12	8–15
Volleyball	7–15	10–18
Weight lifting	5–12	10–18
Wrestling	5–16	—

SOURCE: Adapted from Wilmore, J. H., & Costill, D. L. (1994). *Physiology of sport and exercise.* Champaign, IL: Human Kinetics.

As an upper limit, you should try to be close to the healthy levels of 15% for men and 25% for women. Beyond that, your ideal percentage of body fat is where you perform the best. Attempting to reach an unrealistic body fat percentage can set you back as much as attempting to reach an unrealistic weight.

Assessing Body Composition

The most accurate way to assess body composition is hydrostatic (underwater) weighing. Because muscle is denser than fat (1 pound of muscle takes up the room of 1/3 pound of fat), people with more muscle and less fat will weigh more underwater. Even though there are limitations to hydrostatic weighing, it is referred to as the golden standard because it is the most accurate technique currently available.

Skinfold measurements are the best way to assess body composition when hydrostatic weighing is not available. The rationale behind skinfolds is that there is a relationship between subcutaneous fat and internal fat. Although less accurate than hydrostatic weighing, skinfolds are also useful for determining regional distribution of subcutaneous fat.

Hydrostatic weighing and skinfold measurements must be performed by trained personnel to ensure accuracy. Many sports medicine facilities and universities offer body composition evaluation in addition to $\dot{V}O_{2max}$ testing.

Bioelectrical impedance (a popular technique in health clubs) involves passing a small electrical current throughout the body and measuring the resistance encountered. Lean tissue is a good conductor of electricity; fat is not.

The resistance encountered is inversely related to the amount of lean tissue. Unfortunately, impedance tends to overestimate the body fat of a lean person and underestimate the body fat of an obese person.

Infrared interactance technique uses near-infrared spectroscopy to provide information about the chemical content of the body. A fiberoptic probe is pressed on top of the biceps muscle of the upper arm. A light beam is emitted that penetrates the subcutaneous fat and muscle, which is then reflected off the bone to a silicon detector in the probe. This procedure is only in the early stages of development and its accuracy is questionable.

Body Composition Changes with Exercise

Body weight usually changes very little, if any, in the first few weeks of an exercise program. This is because lean (muscle) weight initially increases at about the same rate that fat weight is being lost. Individuals can become discouraged because the scales show no change, even though body composition (fat versus lean) is changing dramatically. During this time, people should pay more attention to how their clothing fits than what the scale says.

It is even possible to gain weight while losing fat (particularly when including resistance training) because of correspondingly greater muscle gain. For example, a person can gain four pounds of muscle but lose two pounds of fat. This often happens to sedentary women who begin exercising. They may drop two dress sizes but gain two pounds.

Some have even quit exercising when this happens because they're conditioned to go by scale weight.

People who are trying to lose weight should have periodic body composition assessments to measure their fat loss and muscle gain. Your scale weight isn't an accurate indicator of your body composition. And it can't give you the real picture of the changes that you can expect from regular exercise.

14

No Convenient Way to Lose Weight

Permanent Weight Control Is Possible Only Through Lifelong Exercise

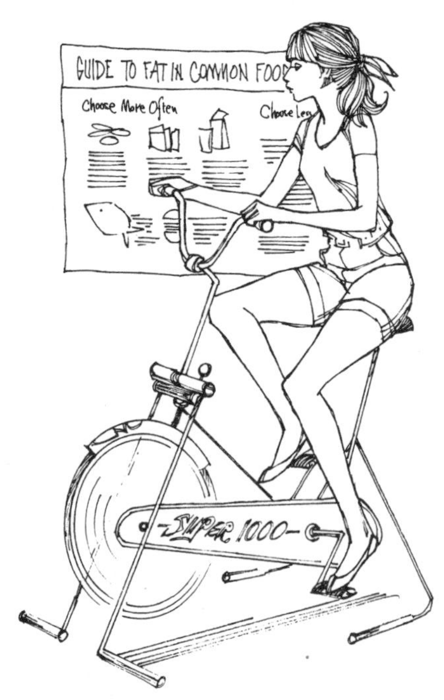

A professional person with a desk job wanted to lose weight. She tried every fad diet but could never keep the pounds off. She tried a sensible diet—well-balanced with a mild calorie deficit—but wasn't happy with her progress.

Finally, a fitness enthusiast got her to walk for 30 minutes a day. She stayed on her diet and slowly lost weight at a rate of about one pound a week. She found that she needed to exercise and eat sensibly to control her weight.

MANY PEOPLE equate weight loss with counting calories. The calories in our food are an important factor in weight control, but as every jaded dieter knows, it's more complicated than that. Exercise is an essential component of a successful weight-control program.

Weight Control and Energy Balance

The energy sources in food, as well as the body's energy expenditure, are measured in units of heat expressed as kilocalories—abbreviated to calories. Protein and carbohydrate both supply 4 calories per gram, fat supplies 9 calories per gram, and alcohol supplies 7 calories per gram.

Weight loss, weight maintenance, or weight gain is all a matter of energy balance. Your body weight will stay the same when your caloric intake equals your caloric expenditure. To lose weight, energy expenditure must be greater than energy intake. To gain weight, energy intake must be greater than energy expenditure. If you want to lose weight, you must eat less, exercise more, or both.

Everyone has a specific requirement for calories. Age, gender, weight, and physical activity determine your caloric needs. The caloric cost of the sport depends on the frequency, intensity, and duration of the activity. The more intense the exercise and the longer it's carried out, the greater will be the caloric cost. Sedentary individuals require about 30 calories per kilogram of body weight daily (14 calories per pound), whereas endurance athletes may require

50 calories per kilogram daily (23 calories per pound) or more. Appendix B lists the caloric expenditure per minute for various activities.

Diet and Body Fat Loss

The American College of Sports Medicine has provided guidelines for desirable weight-loss programs. Adults should consume at least 1,200 calories to meet nutritional requirements. The daily caloric deficit can range from 500 to 1,000 calories, depending on the person's caloric requirement. This mild caloric restriction results in a manageable loss of water, electrolytes, minerals, and fat-free tissue and is less likely to cause malnutrition.

The rate of sustained loss should not exceed one to two pounds per week (3,500 calories equals one pound of fat). Behavior modification techniques should also be used to identify and eliminate eating habits that contribute to intake of excess calories. The lifestyle changes must be realistic because successful weight control requires a lifelong commitment.

Caloric intake can be reduced by eating fewer empty calories—foods high in sugar, fat, and alcohol. Eating habits can also be improved by preparing smaller portions, eating more slowly, and avoiding second helpings. The meal frequency of your diet is also important. Skipping meals earlier in the day is more likely to cause overeating in the evening, so eating regular meals can aid in weight control.

The high–complex carbohydrate, low-fat diet recommended by the Dietary Guidelines for Americans promotes body fat loss for several reasons. Because fat is a concentrated source of calories, reducing fat intake will automatically reduce caloric intake.

Dietary fat is also more fattening than dietary carbohydrate because dietary fat is more likely to be stored as body fat. The conversion of dietary carbohydrate to body fat is metabolically costly—about 23% of the carbohydrate calories are expended in the conversion process. The conversion of dietary fat to body fat is easy and requires little energy—about 3% of the fat calories are expended in the conversion process.

Cutting down on your fat intake does not mean that you can then eat an unlimited amount of carbohydrate and not gain weight. Limiting dietary fat does reduce total calories more than cutting back on dietary carbohydrate, because fat supplies more than twice the calories of carbohydrates by weight. However, if you cut back on fat calories but add calories in the form of carbohydrate calories, you're not going to lose weight. It's a simple matter of energy balance whether you're an athlete or a couch potato.

Exercise and Body Fat Loss

An effective weight-loss regimen incorporates aerobic exercise and resistance training (weight lifting) to reduce fat tissue and preserve lean (muscle) tissue. Aerobic exercise is usually prescribed for weight loss, since the most calories are burned during this type of activity. However, resistance training increases lean weight more than aerobic exercise, and lean weight requires more calories for maintenance than body fat. By increasing the proportion of lean tissue to body fat, both exercises increase the body's calorie-burning ability.

In fact, metabolic rate is closely tied to muscle mass: the greater the muscle mass, the greater the caloric requirement. Changes in body composition toward more muscle mass, along with the actual energy cost of exercising, significantly increase the body's caloric needs.

Caloric restriction causes losses of both body fat and lean tissue. With extreme caloric restrictions, as much as one-third of the weight lost may come from lean tissue. This reduction in muscle mass can significantly reduce caloric needs. In fact, caloric restriction can reduce the resting metabolic rate and caloric expenditure as well, by as much as 15%.

Because dieters need fewer calories, they lose less weight. This commonly leads to the plateau phase, when weight loss slows or even ceases. Dieters often become frustrated and end their caloric restriction. When the resting metabolic rate drops, caloric intake must be reduced by the same amount to maintain weight loss—a demanding situation for even the most dedicated dieter.

The metabolic rate may remain elevated after moderate exercise (60% of $\dot{V}O_{2max}$) lasting 40 minutes or longer. However, these added calories equal only about 5% to 6% of the total caloric cost of the activity. This increased caloric expenditure, over and above the energy cost of the exercise itself, is unlikely to have any real effect on weight loss.

Combining exercise with caloric restriction can counteract the decrease in metabolic rate that occurs with caloric restriction. Exercise also reduces the loss of lean tissue experienced with caloric restriction. And combining diet and exercise promotes faster body fat loss than using either alone.

Exercise Recommendations to Lose Body Fat

People who want to lose body fat should include aerobic exercise 3 to 5 days per week, for 30 to 60 minutes, at 60% to 90% of maximal heart rate (50% to 85% of $\dot{V}O_{2max}$). Increased exercise frequency and duration (5 days a week for 60 minutes) are associated with greater fat losses from increased caloric expenditure. Resistance training should be included several times per week.

The goal is to expend 300 calories per exercise session for a total weekly caloric expenditure of at least 1,000 calories per week, since this seems to represent a threshold for body fat loss. In practical terms, 300 calories is roughly equal to what a person will use in jogging three miles, walking four miles, swimming one mile, bicycling twelve miles, or participating in an aerobics class (including warm-up and cool-down).

The exercise intensity should be lower for an individual with a low initial level of fitness. Low- to moderate-intensity exercise is recommended for overweight people who are just beginning to exercise. High-intensity exercise is associated with an increased risk of orthopedic injuries. Also, unfit people who engage in high-intensity exercise usually find it unpleasant and may stop exercising altogether.

The only drawback of low-intensity exercise is that the person must exercise longer to burn off the calories. Other than that, a low-intensity workout that expends 300 calories in one hour is just as beneficial for body fat loss as a high-intensity workout that expends 300 calories in 30 minutes.

Although body fat can also be reduced through anaerobic exercise like sprinting or interval training, the exercise usually doesn't last long enough to achieve a caloric deficit comparable to that realized with aerobic exercise. Most people who use anaerobic workouts are trying to increase their speed rather than lose body fat.

Misconceptions About Exercise

Some people believe that exercise will increase their appetite and food intake, thereby offsetting the calories expended during exercise. When you consider the effect of exercise on food intake, you must account for the intensity and duration of activity. Obviously, athletes who spend many hours in vigorous training each day have high calorie intakes, but they also have low percentages of body fat. Sedentary people tend to eat more than people who engage in light to moderate activity for up to an hour each day. Exercise within this range appears to be a mild appetite suppressant.

Another common misconception is that it takes a tremendous amount of exercise to lose body fat. For example, you may hear that you have to run 35 miles to lose one pound of fat. However, the calorie-expending effects of each exercise session add up. A 3,500 calorie deficit equals one pound of fat, whether this happens rapidly or gradually over a period of time. Patience pays off, because this kind of gradual weight loss is more permanent than rapid weight loss.

Spot Reduction

If you hope to spot reduce, you're in for disappointment. Exercise, even when localized, draws from all the fat stores of the body, not just from the local fat deposits. Tennis players, for example, have been found to have the same triceps skinfold on both arms, even though their dominant arm was exercised more.

Exercising a specific area does increase muscle tone and may make the person look thinner. For example, substantial reductions in abdominal girth can result from localized exercise such as sit-ups. This is not due to fat loss. Rather, the abdominal muscles are strengthened and better able to hold in the abdomen.

Spot reduction to eliminate so-called cellulite from specific areas of the body is vigorously promoted by creators of creams, wraps, and special exercise equipment. Cellulite doesn't exist; it's just a gimmicky name for subcutaneous fat that has a dimpled appearance. Stay away from any sales pitch that uses the term. The only way to get rid of fat deposits is through diet and exercise, and there is no way any cream or device can reduce fat on one part of the body.

The Fat-Burning Myth

We know that fat makes its greatest energy contribution during low- to moderate-intensity exercise. This knowledge has led to recommendations that individuals who want to lose weight should exercise at a lower intensity.

The concept of fat-burning versus carbohydrate-burning

exercises is a common misconception. Some believe that individuals who want to lose body fat should exercise at a lower intensity, as fat contributes more to the metabolic mixture at this level. Unfortunately, this assumption misses the whole point: Regular exercise is beneficial for weight loss because it creates a prolonged caloric deficit.

The fuel being burned to create this caloric deficit (fat or carbohydrate) is not important. There is no scientific evidence that using fat as fuel will produce greater body fat loss than using carbohydrate as fuel. It is the caloric deficit that is important.

For example, it is doubtful that a runner would lose more body fat by jogging five miles slowly than by running five miles at race pace. Although fat contributes more calories during jogging than racing, both activities burn the same amount of calories and so have the same effect on body fat.

Although a greater percentage of fat may be burned with low-intensity exercise, the total amount of fat burned may be greater with high-intensity exercise because the total energy expenditure is higher during intense activity. The fuel burned during exercise (carbohydrate or fat) doesn't matter when the goal is to lose weight.

In other words, low-intensity exercise uses a greater percentage of fat than high-intensity exercise, but the fat calories (and carbohydrate calories) are being burned at a relatively slow rate—4 to 5 calories per minute.

By comparison, high-intensity exercise uses a smaller percentage of fat, but this smaller percentage (along with carbohydrate) is burned at a much higher rate—10 to 15 calories per minute. Thus, the total amount of fat burned may be greater at the higher-intensity levels.

Many individuals have confused the proportion of fat used as fuel with the more important rate of fuel utilization, which is a key concept in exercise-induced body fat loss. When the goal of an exercise program is to lose weight, the exercise should create a caloric deficit. To lose one pound of body fat, an individual must expend 3,500 calories, whether those calories come from fat or carbohydrate.

Keep in mind that the decreased number of calories burned during low-intensity exercise may be detrimental for fit people trying to lose body fat. If the fit person's food intake stays the same and the exercise time isn't increased to compensate for the reduced caloric expenditure of low-intensity exercise, the result may be a slow but steady weight gain!

Focus on Body Fat Percentage

A healthy percentage of body fat for men and women is 15% and 25%, respectively. If you are overweight (because of a large muscle mass) but not overfat, relax. If you are overweight and overfat, combine mild to moderate calorie restriction with an aerobic exercise and resistance training program. This combination will promote body fat loss. If you're overfat but not overweight (because of a small muscle mass), skip the diet and shape up with aerobic exercise and resistance training.

15

Running on Empty

The Dangers of Starvation by Choice

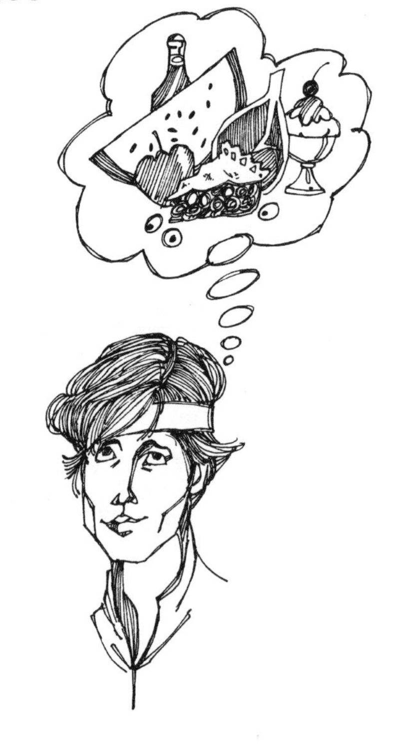

A man who took up cycling became more interested in his overall health and ate less red meat. From there, he decided that fasting would cleanse his body and help him to feel even healthier.

The day before a 200-mile ride he fasted. After 50 miles of the ride he was desperate for food, begging some nourishment from his riding partners. His performance that day was much slower than usual. However, he claimed that fasting "enhanced his experience."

He continued fasting, although his performance kept deteriorating.

STARVATION IS IN. Whether we want to look like fashion models or improve our performance, we are prey to a multitude of misconceptions—from bizarre diet regimens to eating disorders. These practices can harm performance and have serious health consequences.

Low-Carbohydrate Fad Diets

Like so many other people, athletes often search for a quick and easy way to lose weight. Fad diets are popular because they usually promise the dieter rapid weight loss.

Fad diets are usually low in carbohydrate and cause muscle and liver glycogen depletion. Because water is stored with glycogen, a large amount of water is lost on these diets. Dieters cherish this rapid weight loss and assume that it represents fat loss. Actually, their body fat stores are virtually untouched. And, as the body adjusts for the water deficit, the weight loss slows or ceases. The dieter often becomes frustrated and abandons the diet.

Complications associated with low-carbohydrate diets include ketosis, hypoglycemia, calcium depletion, weakness, nausea, electrolyte loss, gout, and possible kidney problems. Vitamin and mineral deficiencies are other potential problems on such unbalanced diets. In addition, low-carbohydrate diets are usually high in fat and may increase the risk of heart disease when used repeatedly.

The Zone Diet

This popular fad diet revolves around the myth that high-carbohydrate diets make people fat and impair athletic performance. Supposedly, to "burn body fat" and "reach your optimum athletic performance," you must eat the "perfect ratio" of 40% carbohydrate, 30% protein, and 30% fat at each meal and snack.

A high-carbohydrate diet does not make you fat. It's your total caloric intake that's important. You have to eat too many calories to lay down body fat, not just a lot of calories from carbohydrate. Carbohydrates will be converted to fat only if they are eaten in excess. And, compared to dietary fat, dietary carbohydrate is more likely to be burned for energy than stored as fat.

The Zone diet doesn't help you burn more fat or change your body's preference for carbohydrates over fat as fuel. The best way to crank up your body's fat-burning ability is to keep working out. And as for gradual loss of body fat, that comes from burning more calories than you take in, not from some special dietary ratio.

Fasting

Occasionally even fasting is used for weight loss. Some proponents recommend fasting for body fat loss or to eliminate "toxins." From a physiological standpoint, fasting fails on all accounts.

A prolonged fast can cause anemia, impaired kidney and liver function, kidney stones, low blood pressure, and mineral imbalances. After a week-long fast, as much as one-third of the weight lost may come from lean tissue. Deaths from prolonged fasting have occurred, usually in people who believed this would "purify" their body or cure them of some disease.

Fasting is ineffective as a weight-loss diet because it decreases the body's metabolic rate. The large initial weight loss associated with fasting is actually water loss from muscle and liver glycogen depletion. When the person resumes eating, glycogen and water stores are replaced and body weight is regained.

The only things that are "cleansed" from the body are the minerals needed for muscle contractions, nerve transmissions, and the regulation of body fluids. Though fat, protein, and carbohydrate stores can provide energy for a period of time, the body needs the vitamins and minerals supplied by food to metabolize these fuel stores and carry on necessary physiological functions.

Effects on Performance

Fad diets and fasting are especially unsuitable for athletes and individuals who exercise regularly. Because muscle glycogen is the preferred fuel for most types of exercise, low-carbohydrate diets impair a person's ability to exercise by reducing muscle glycogen stores. These diets also make active people more susceptible to hypoglycemia because of insufficient liver glycogen stores.

Athletes who follow a fad diet or fast are likely to feel irritable as a result of inadequate dietary carbohydrate and the subsequent ketosis that results from fat breakdown. Ketosis can also cause nausea and central nervous system depression. The accompanying symptoms—sluggishness, loss of coordination, inability to concentrate—are incompatible with optimum exercise performance. Last, dehydration and electrolyte losses impair body temperature regulation and increase the risk of heat illnesses.

Body fat loss can be accomplished far more effectively and healthfully with exercise and a low-fat diet. Furthermore, fad diets and fasting can be very dangerous for individuals with chronic medical conditions such as diabetes, coronary heart disease, and liver or kidney disease.

What Fad Diets Don't Teach

Fad diets and fasting are also faulty from a behavioral standpoint because they tend to reinforce bad habits once the dieters return to their usual eating habits. Dieters are also distracted from the truth that real, long-term weight control requires fundamental changes in lifestyle.

The dieter is not encouraged to learn about the composition, planning, and preparation of foods so as to make well-educated food selections. Rather, most fad diets establish rigid rules and limitations that can be followed only for a short time. Typically, the dieter then abandons the diet and the weight is regained.

Fad diets appeal to the emotions and therefore perpetuate the myth that weight loss can be achieved quickly and easily. Rarely do they address the true need to make basic changes in lifelong ways of looking at and dealing with food. But the greatest danger associated with these regimens is that the diet will be nutritionally unbalanced and have harmful side effects.

Evaluating Weight-Loss Programs

"Miraculous" diets tend to produce only miraculous profits for their promoters. They are all based on the false hope that a magic combination of foods and/or supplements can cause weight loss independent of calories. Believers are more likely to lose dollars than pounds. When evaluating a weight-loss program, you should consider the following points:

1. Does the diet include a variety of foods from the Food Guide Pyramid to ensure nutritional adequacy? Or does it suggest that a certain food is either the *key* to weight loss or the primary *villain* that keeps people overweight? Be wary of diets that eliminate certain foods entirely or promote eating them in "special fat-burning combinations."
2. Does the program avoid sensational claims such as "revolutionary," "miraculous," "quick and easy," "metabolically proven," "eat all you want," "burns fat and builds muscle," and "100% success rate"?
3. Is the diet's effectiveness well documented by research published in credible scientific journals (consult a registered dietitian) and not based on

testimonials by famous people or self-proclaimed experts?

4. Does it include modification of eating patterns and exercise?
5. Does it avoid the use of diuretics and/or appetite suppressants?

Ineffective Weight-Loss Aids

Vibrating belts are completely ineffective; such passive exercise doesn't increase a person's calorie expenditure and can't break up fat. Similarly, body wraps and elastic belts can't melt away fat. Electric muscle stimulators can cause specific muscles to contract, but they have no effect on fat deposits. All these gimmicks may *appear* to work by causing temporary water loss or muscle contraction. Although the person may look thinner for a short time, only the person's wallet experiences permanent shrinkage.

Thigh creams containing aminophyllin (an asthma drug) are the latest dubious treatment for female "thunder thighs." One study showed that applying the thigh cream for 6 weeks caused an average loss of one-half inch—an almost undetectable change. The thigh creams that are sold contain less aminophyllin than used in the study, and their long-term safety and effectiveness are questionable.

Nonprescription diet pills, especially herbal products, are the most popular fraudulent weight-loss product. Herbal products often have strong drug and/or toxic effects and are especially dangerous because they vary in potency. Pills that contain ephedrine or ma huang (a stimulant similar to amphetamine) can be extremely hazardous. An ephedrine overdose, which is common with diet pills, can cause a rapid heart rate, an irregular heart rhythm, and even death.

Wearing rubber suits, plastic suits, or heavy clothing during exercise to "melt away" fat is also dangerous and ineffective. The weight loss is from fluid, not fat. And this apparel prevents the evaporation of sweat, which is necessary to reduce body temperature. Dehydration, heat illness, and even heat stroke may be the result. Lounging in a sauna will also cause weight loss from sweating. Of course, the weight will return to normal when the sweat-induced water loss is replaced.

Eating Disorders

Almost all active people are concerned about their weight. Ideally, this concern will spur them to achieve ideal body composition for health and performance. Instead, some athletes can become obsessed with achieving an ideal weight or lean appearance. As a result, they may develop disordered eating behaviors that jeopardize both performance and health. Awareness of these life-threatening disorders is growing, but diagnosis and treatment lag far behind the problem.

Eating disorders are severe disturbances in eating behavior. *Anorexia nervosa* is characterized by a person's refusal to maintain body weight at or above a minimally normal weight for age and height; a distorted body image (the person feels fat even when emaciated); an intense fear of gaining weight or becoming fat although the person is obviously underweight; and amenorrhea (the absence of at least three consecutive menstrual cycles).

Bulimia nervosa is characterized by binge eating (rapid consumption of large amounts of food in a short period of time) followed by inappropriate compensatory behavior to prevent weight gain. This behavior can involve self-induced vomiting, misuse of laxatives, diuretics, enemas, fasting, or excessive exercise. The binge eating and inappropriate compensatory behaviors both occur at least twice a week for at least 3 months, and self-evaluation is unduly influenced by body shape and weight.

The term *anorexia athletica* is used to identify athletes who show significant symptoms of eating disorders but who do not meet the criteria for anorexia nervosa or bulimia nervosa. The classic features of anorexia athletica are an intense fear of weight gain or becoming fat even though the individual is lean; weight loss accomplished by a reduction in energy intake (often combined with exercise); and restrictive energy intake below that required to maintain high training volume. Binge eating is common and such athletes frequently use pathogenic methods of weight control such as vomiting, laxatives, and diuretics.

Female athletes are at greater risk for eating disorders than are female nonathletes or males. The risk is highest in endurance sports (distance running and swimming), appearance sports (gymnastics, figure skating, diving, ballet, and body building), and weight classification sports (wrestling and lightweight crew). The prevalence of eating disorders may be as great as 50% in these high-risk sports.

Athletes in high-risk sports may have weight loss and

dietary behaviors similar to those of people with eating disorders. When an athlete develops an obsession with food and fatness, it is often difficult to tell whether the obsession is due to the belief that "thin will win," or if there is a true eating disorder. It's important to distinguish between behaviors associated with requirements of the sport and the existence of an actual eating disorder.

Warning Signs

Table 15-1 presents a list of warning signs for anorexia nervosa and bulimia nervosa. These do not signify that an eating disorder exists, but they justify further evaluation by a

TABLE 15-1
WARNING SIGNS FOR ANOREXIA NERVOSA AND BULIMIA NERVOSA (NCAA)

WARNING SIGNS FOR ANOREXIA NERVOSA	WARNING SIGNS FOR BULIMIA NERVOSA
• Dramatic loss in weight	• Noticeable weight loss or gain
• A preoccupation with food, calories, and weight	• Excessive concern about weight
• Wearing baggy or layered clothing	• Bathroom visits after meals
• Relentless, excessive exercise	• Depressive moods
• Mood swings	• Strict dieting followed by eating binges
• Avoiding food-related social activities	• Increasing criticism of one's body

Note: The presence of one or two of these signs does not necessarily indicate the presence of an eating disorder. Absolute diagnosis should be done by appropriate professionals.

SOURCE: National Collegiate Athletic Association, Kansas City, MO, 1990.

health professional. Recognizing the signs of eating disorders helps to facilitate early diagnosis and treatment.

People suspected of having an eating disorder should be approached privately by someone they trust. If the person is not receptive, he or she will at least know where to turn for help in the future. Ideally, the person should be referred to a physician, psychologist, registered dietitian, or health care team who specialize in treating eating disorders. Eating disorders are considered addictive disorders and are very difficult to treat.

Although it is not easy to talk to someone about the possible presence of an eating disorder, ignoring the problem only increases the danger to the person. The physiological consequences of eating disorders are considerable and can include death. Getting treatment is also the only way to preserve athletic prowess. Eating disorders threaten performance as well as health.

Complications of anorexia and/or bulimia may include malnutrition, electrolyte imbalances, dehydration, gastrointestinal problems, cardiac irregularities, organ damage, fainting, and seizures. Growth in adolescents may decrease as the duration of the disorder increases and lead to a shorter adult stature. Bulimics can develop dental erosion and decay due to repeated vomiting of highly acidic gastric content. In severe cases of anorexia, individuals who cannot overcome their aversion to eating may eventually starve to death.

When an eating disorder is detected, the athlete should not be allowed to compete until she or he is under treatment. If the disorder remains untreated, the person may suffer permanent physical injury. An athlete will often deny the significance of an injury and keep exercising, thereby causing more damage.

Sources of Help

Many professionals specializing in this area recommend that people who have eating disorders join eating disorder self-help groups to receive peer support, newsletters, and other help. These are nonprofit organizations and appreciate requests for information that are accompanied by a self-addressed, stamped, business-size envelope. Among the most popular organizations are these:

- American Anorexia/Bulimia Association, Inc.
  418 East 76th Street, New York, NY 10021
  (212) 734-1114
- National Association of Anorexia Nervosa & Associated Disorders, Inc. (ANAD)
  P.O. Box 271, Highland Park, IL 60035
  (708) 831-3438
- Anorexia Nervosa and Related Eating Disorders (ANRED)
  P.O. Box 5102, Eugene, OR 97405
  (541) 344-1144
- National Anorexic Aid Society (NAAS)
  5796 Karl Road, Columbus, OH 43229
  (614) 436-1112

16

Sports Nutrition Quackery

Keep Your Hand on Your Wallet

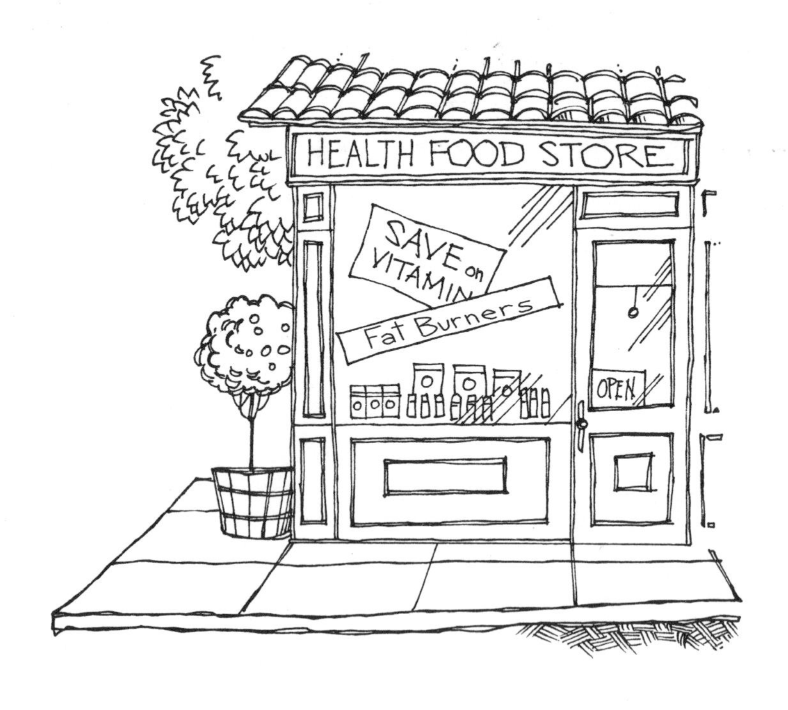

A woman runner was training 70 miles a week for a marathon, which she hoped to finish in 2 hours and 55 minutes—a goal within her reach.

Her well-meaning coach had her follow a diet containing 40% carbohydrate, 30% protein, and 30% fat the week before the marathon. He thought this would help her burn more fat and thereby improve her endurance.

She felt good the morning of the run and ran well for the first quarter of the marathon. As she pushed onto the 13-mile mark, though, her legs felt heavy and slow. She hit the wall and struggled to finish, relying mainly on her form, which was very good.

She had trained twice as many miles for this marathon, but failed to improve her time. If it hadn't been for her natural ability, she probably wouldn't even have finished.

WE WANT TO BELIEVE. Even when we've signed up for that magic powder, new wonder diet, new dietary supplement again and again—and been disappointed again and again—we're ready for the next hustle. If we're lucky, it only costs us money, and perhaps some missed trophies.

Nutrition Quackery

"New endurance performance breakthrough! Makes more oxygen available to your muscles. Increases your aerobic capacity without additional training. Our unique supplement is an oxygen-releasing substance extracted from natural foods by a secret process. Send $49.95 for your starter capsules now!"

Sounds too good to be true? It is.

If you read a typical fitness magazine, you know there is no shortage of nutrition supplements that supposedly increase speed, enhance endurance, relieve muscle soreness, improve muscle mass, or reduce body fat. Some advertisements even claim their wonder product does all the above.

Athletes seek that secret ingredient that will enhance their workout and give them the edge over their competitors. As a result, they are susceptible to nutrition quackery.

Nutrition quacks promote false and/or unproven nutrition products or services for a profit. Quacks can be sincere and misguided individuals as well as charlatans and frauds. Quackery is successful because we want to believe in something magical that can improve performance more than hard training or a prudent diet.

You can avoid being a victim of a nutrition rip-off by learning to recognize the techniques used by nutrition quacks to manipulate consumers. When you observe any of the following, stop, take a deep breath, and keep your hand on your wallet.

Warning Signs

The claims sound too good to be true, but they are what people want to hear. Nutrition quackery is successful because quacks play on emotions and misinformation. Most of us want to believe that there are mystical ways to improve our performance that can bypass the rigors of training and diet. However, we are rarely told of possible side effects or other harm that might result from the promoted product or dietary regimen.

Quacks also encourage distrust of reputable health professionals such as medical doctors, registered dietitians, and other nutrition scientists. They ridicule the nutrient content of our food supply and claim that the foods we need to meet nutritional requirements can't be purchased in grocery stores. They refer to their unproven treatments as true alternatives to reputable medical care. Although choices do exist among current legitimate treatments, the alternatives promoted by quacks are usually ineffective and/or unsafe.

Quacks often use case histories, testimonials, and subjective evidence to justify their exaggerated claims. Quacks try to appear trustworthy by having well-known athletes promote their product. Testimonial evidence is by definition biased and unreliable. Scientists report their studies in reputable journals, and their work is reviewed and evaluated by other scientists prior to publication. Controlled experiments that can be confirmed by repetition are the best way to document the truth of the information.

Evaluating Claims

You need to be discriminating about the nutrition information you read and hear. Most victims of nutrition fraud aren't gullible, only unsuspecting. Magazines, books, and the media overflow with medical advice—some reliable, some inaccurate. Here are some guidelines you can use to evaluate nutrition claims:

What are the qualifications of the person recommending the product or diet? A reputable person usually has a background or current affiliation with an accredited university or medical school offering programs in the fields of nutrition or medicine. Beware the title *nutritionist.* It can be used by anyone, regardless of training. Even Ph.D. is no guarantee. Sad to say, a quack can purchase the credential from a diploma mill (an unaccredited institution) to appear legitimate.

What evidence does the person supply for any claims that are made? The claims should be supported with references to the scientific journals that published the original research. Is the information factual and specific or vague and highly emotional? Are the recommendations based on published scientific evidence or on personal testimonials?

If the information is written, why was it published? Is someone trying to sell you something? Does the material encourage gradual changes in your lifestyle, or does it promise to dramatically enhance performance or guarantee fast results? Does the author recommend eating a variety of foods, or are certain foods eliminated? Are expensive supplements recommended as the only way to ensure nutritional adequacy?

Do the suggestions appear to agree with most recommendations of medical and sports science professionals? Professional journals and newsletters review articles in a wide range of lay publications and judge their credibility. If you don't have access to these—and most athletes don't—you can seek the advice of a registered dietitian (R.D.) or other qualified nutrition professional at a local university, health department, or hospital. If you're considering big changes in eating habits that have kept you healthy and performing well until now, this extra digging is worthwhile.

Other Strategies Quacks Use

Quacks are very clever at imitating actual health professionals and scientists. When quacks assess a person's nutritional status, they use various "tests" to diagnose nutritional deficiencies and food allergies. They use these tests to appear scientific, convince people to buy nutrition supplements, or even to profit directly from the cost of the test. The tests used by quacks include applied kinesiology, live cell analysis, iridology, hair analysis, and cytotoxic testing.

Using fake tests, these fake nutritionists always find something wrong. Their typical diagnoses include food allergies, hypoglycemia, malabsorption, glandular disturbances, adrenal insufficiency, trace vitamin and mineral deficiencies, and the buildup of various toxins in the body. These are all problems that sound ominous and are difficult to prove or disprove.

Quacks may claim they are doing a nutrition assessment —but what makes up a valid nutrition assessment? A nutrition assessment may be part of a general health examination and requires the combined expertise of a medical doctor and a registered dietitian. It generally includes medical history, dietary history, and clinical evaluations. If neither a registered dietitian nor a physician is involved, you should be suspicious.

Quackery is very subtle. It plays on athletes' longing to find something that will give them an edge. In many events the difference between winning and losing is in divisions of seconds, so it is not surprising that athletes are susceptible to claims for magical foods or nutrients. The placebo effect by itself is powerful enough to produce beneficial results. When athletes are convinced that certain products improve performance, their belief may enable them to perform better, even though there is nothing useful in the product. Just because a friend may ride the placebo effect to a better performance, it doesn't mean you will.

Most of the time, quacks only do injury to our wallets and hopes, promising benefits they can't deliver.

However, they can cause real harm when necessary medical treatment is delayed at a time when it could be most effective in treating an illness or injury.

Ergogenic Aids

Ergogenic aids represent the trendiest area in sports nutrition. They supposedly enhance performance above levels anticipated under normal conditions. Ergogenic means "work producing." Many athletes believe that certain ergogenic aids will give them a competitive edge. In fact, many offer no benefits, and some are actually harmful.

For several reasons, athletes believe that various products have helped them. The use of the product often coincides with natural improvement as a result of training. Also, increased self-confidence or a placebo effect inspires greater performance. This psychological benefit should be weighed against the dangers of misinformation, wasted money, misplaced faith, and adverse side effects that can result from use of some of these products.

Currently popular ergogenic aids include the following:

Antioxidant vitamins (C, E, and beta-carotene).

Claim: Protect against exercise-induced muscle damage due to free-radical production.

Fact: May protect against muscle damage following prolonged endurance exercise but do not improve performance. In the small quantities found in food, these antioxidants help to stop the production and spread of harmful free-radical chain reactions. In the high amounts found in supplements, they may actually increase the production of free radicals.

Carnitine (a compound synthesized in the body from the amino acids lysine and methionine).

Claim: Increases fat metabolism and decreases body fat.

Fact: Carnitine facilitates the transfer of fatty acids into the mitochondria (the energy powerhouses of the cell) where they are burned for fuel in the aerobic energy system. There is no evidence that carnitine supplementation increases the use of fatty acids during exercise, or decreases body fat. There is no dietary requirement for carnitine.

Choline (precursor of the neurotransmitter acetylcholine and of lecithin, a substance involved in fat transport).

Claim: Increases strength (by increasing acetylcholine) and decreases body fat (by increasing lecithin).

Fact: There is no dietary requirement for this substance and a deficiency has never been demonstrated in humans. The body can manufacture choline from methionine, an essential amino acid. There is no evidence that increasing choline intake will increase strength or decrease body fat.

Chromium (an active component of the glucose tolerance factor, which facilitates the action of insulin).

Claim: Increases muscle mass, decreases body fat, and promotes weight loss.

Fact: The researcher who holds the patent on chromium picolinate claims that it increases muscle mass and decreases body fat. Unfortunately, patenting laws do not require that claims for health products be valid. A huge amount of independent research indicates that chromium picolinate has no effect on muscle mass, body fat, or weight loss.

Coenzyme Q10 (a catalyst in the aerobic energy system).

Claim: Optimizes ATP production to increase energy and stamina.

Fact: There is no dietary requirement for this substance and a deficiency has never been demonstrated in humans. Supplementation with coenzyme Q10 does not improve endurance performance or aerobic capacity.

Ginseng (extract of ginseng root).

Claim: Increases energy, increases resistance to stress and disease, and cures almost everything.

Fact: No other drug has all the healthful properties that are attributed to ginseng. The existence of a genuine cure-all is unlikely. Until proper research is conducted, the claims for ginseng are not valid. Because it is expensive, the commercial preparations may contain little or no ginseng. The best-documented side effects of ginseng are insomnia, and to a lesser extent, diarrhea and skin eruptions; however, the prolonged use of ginseng appears to be relatively safe.

Inosine (a nucleoside involved in the formation of purines).

Claim: Increases ATP production, increases strength, and enhances recovery.

Fact: There are no performance benefits from consuming inosine. Inosine is broken down during digestion and does not reach the body's cells intact.

Lecithin (phosphatidylcholine).

Claim: Prevents fat gain.

Fact: Lecithin is a phospholipid. Phospholipids are powerful emulsifying agents and so are essential for the digestion and absorption of fat. Although lecithin has a role in the digestion of dietary fat, it has no effect on body fat. The body produces an ample amount of lecithin and supplementation is unnecessary.

Lipotropic factors (includes carnitine, coenzyme Q10, arginine, and ornithine).

Claim: Increases fat loss with exercise.

Fact: See comments under appropriate sections.

Metabolic bars (such as PR Bar).

Claim: Eating metabolic bars and following a strict dietary regimen (40% carbohydrate, 30% protein, and 30% fat) increases fat metabolism and promotes body fat loss.

Fact: There is no evidence that metabolic bars improve fat metabolism or decrease body fat above and beyond the effects of exercise training. Athletes who follow the dietary regimen may have impaired performance due to low muscle glycogen stores.

Omega-3 fatty acids (polyunsaturated fatty acids found mostly in fish oils).

Claim: Stimulates release of growth hormone.

Fact: Omega-3 fatty acids may be converted to prostaglandins (hormone-like substances) in the body. A specific prostaglandin called PGE 1 does stimulate growth hormone release. There is no proof that omega-3 fatty acids improve aerobic endurance or strength.

Succinate (a metabolite in the aerobic energy system).

Claim: Enhances metabolism, reduces lactic acid, and maintains ATP production.

Fact: Succinate is an intermediary in the aerobic pathway. Supplemental succinate will not speed up the process of aerobic metabolism or ATP production as this is controlled by enzymes within the pathway.

Superoxide dismutase (enzyme).

Claim: Protects the body against oxidative cell damage incurred from aerobic metabolism.

Fact: Superoxide dismutase is an antioxidant enzyme found in most body cells. It works with other antioxidants such as vitamin C and E to protect the cells from oxidation. No benefit for humans has ever been demonstrated. This is because oral superoxide dismutase is digested and does not reach the bloodstream intact.

The Bottom Line

New ergogenic aids for athletes are constantly emerging. These products are often marketed without any supportive scientific research to indicate the potential benefits or possible harmful side effects. Prosecutions or other legal actions take years, and the promoter can reap huge profits during the delay.

Under our consumer protection laws, *a substance is considered a drug if a medical claim is made for it,* even though it is a food or dietary supplement. However, just about anything can be sold as long as it is called a dietary supplement. Because the Food and Drug Administration cannot regulate dietary supplements, these products are not evaluated for safety and effectiveness.

Although claims on the label cannot be false or misleading, supplement manufacturers often use advertising techniques such as testimonials and pamphlets that are protected by the first amendment to the Constitution (freedom of speech). People often believe that magazine, radio, and television ads and testimonials are proof of effectiveness.

The supplement manufacturers currently have the advantage: Their products don't have to be safe or effective. People tend to believe that the products on the market have been researched, tested, and inspected. Avoid buying products with bogus claims like "fat burner," "fat metabolizer," "energy enhancer," "performance booster," "strength booster," "ergogenic aid," "anabolic optimizer," and "genetic optimizer."

Your best protection against nutrition fraud is to be an informed consumer. If you have questions about a particular supplement, contact a registered dietitian specializing in sports nutrition or the National Council Against Health Fraud, P. O. Box 1276, Loma Linda, CA 92354.

True Scientific Advantages

We know there are definite ways to improve endurance—using carbohydrate loading; maintaining proper hydration; consuming carbohydrate before, during, and after prolonged exercise; consuming caffeine before prolonged exercise; and most important, eating a well-balanced diet rich in complex carbohydrates.

Many factors are responsible for performance, and scientific research continues to identify these variables. Valid nutrition concepts are built on such evidence, not rash claims. As researchers continue to investigate fuel usage during exercise, and the effects of food and fluid intake for such exercise, we can continue to improve endurance. To me, that's exciting!

Appendix A

Professional Organizations

The following groups specialize in health, nutrition, and exercise issues.

- **American College of Sports Medicine (ACSM)**
  401 West Michigan St.
  Indianapolis, IN 46202-3233
  (317) 637-9200
  Online: http://www.acsm.org/sportsmed
  Publication: Medicine and Science in Sports and Exercise
  Purpose: To communicate research on exercise to members and public
  Membership: People in fields of exercise and medicine

- **American Dietetic Association (ADA)**
  216 West Jackson Blvd.
  Chicago, IL 60606-6995
  (312) 899-0040
  Online: http://www.eatright.org/
  Publication: Journal of the American Dietetic Association
  Purpose: To promote optimal health, nutrition, and well-being
  Membership: Dietitians who are members of the American Dietetic Association

- **ADA Practice Group of Sports, Cardiovascular, and Wellness Nutritionists (SCAN)**
  7730 Belleview, #G6
  Englewood, CO 80111
  (303) 779-1950
  Purpose: To promote integration of nutrition and exercise

Appendix B

Caloric Expenditures

The following table lists approximate caloric expenditures per minute for various physical activities.

SOURCE: Adapted from Williams, M. H. (1992). *Nutrition for fitness and sport*, 3rd ed. Dubuque, IA: William C. Brown.

Appendix B

Approximate Caloric Expenditure Per Minute For Various Physical Activities

Body Weight in Kilograms	45	50	55	59	64	68	73	77	82	86	91	95	100
Body Weight in Pounds	100	110	120	130	140	150	160	170	180	190	200	210	220
Sedentary Activities													
Lying quietly	.99	1.1	1.2	1.3	1.4	1.5	1.6	1.7	1.8	1.9	2.0	2.1	2.2
Sitting and writing	1.2	1.4	1.5	1.7	1.8	1.9	2.0	2.2	2.3	2.4	2.5	2.7	2.8
Standing with light work	2.7	3.0	3.3	3.5	3.8	4.1	4.4	4.6	4.9	5.2	5.4	5.7	6.0
Physical Activities													
Archery	3.1	3.5	3.8	4.1	4.5	4.8	5.1	5.4	5.7	6.0	6.4	6.7	7.0
Badminton													
Recreational singles	3.6	4.0	4.4	4.7	5.1	5.4	5.8	6.2	6.6	6.9	7.3	7.6	8.0
Competitive	5.9	6.4	7.0	7.6	8.2	8.8	9.4	10.0	10.6	11.2	11.8	12.4	13.0
Baseball													
Player	3.1	3.4	3.8	4.1	4.4	4.7	5.0	5.3	5.6	5.9	6.3	6.6	6.9
Pitcher	3.9	4.3	4.7	5.1	5.5	5.9	6.3	6.7	7.1	7.4	7.9	8.2	8.6
Basketball													
Recreational	4.9	5.5	6.0	6.5	7.0	7.5	8.0	8.5	9.0	9.5	10.0	10.5	11.0
Vigorous competition	6.5	7.2	7.8	8.5	9.2	9.9	10.5	11.2	11.9	12.5	13.2	13.8	14.5

Appendix B *(continued)*

Approximate Caloric Expenditure Per Minute For Various Physical Activities

Body Weight in Kilograms		45	50	55	59	64	68	73	77	82	86	91	95	100
Body Weight in Pounds		100	110	120	130	140	150	160	170	180	190	200	210	220
Bicycling, level														
(mph)	(min/mile)													
5	12:00	1.9	2.1	2.3	2.5	2.7	2.9	3.1	3.3	3.5	3.7	3.9	4.1	4.3
10	6:00	4.2	4.6	5.1	5.5	5.9	6.4	6.8	7.2	7.6	8.1	8.5	8.9	9.4
15	4:00	7.3	8.0	8.7	9.5	10.0	10.9	11.6	12.4	13.1	13.8	14.5	15.3	16.0
20	3:00	10.7	11.7	12.8	13.9	14.9	16.0	17.1	18.1	19.2	20.3	21.3	22.4	23.5
Canoeing														
(mph)	(min/mile)													
2.5	24	1.9	2.1	2.3	2.5	2.7	2.9	3.1	3.3	3.5	3.7	3.9	4.1	4.3
4.0	15	4.4	4.9	5.3	5.8	6.2	6.7	7.1	7.6	8.0	8.5	8.9	9.4	9.8
5.0	12	5.7	6.3	6.9	7.5	8.1	8.7	9.3	9.8	10.4	11.0	11.6	12.2	12.8
Dancing														
Moderately (waltz)		3.1	3.5	3.8	4.1	4.5	4.8	5.1	5.4	5.7	6.0	6.4	6.7	7.0
Active (square, disco)		4.5	5.0	5.4	5.9	6.3	6.8	7.3	7.7	8.2	8.6	9.1	9.5	10.0
Aerobic (vigorously)		6.0	6.7	7.3	7.9	8.5	9.1	9.7	10.3	10.9	11.5	12.1	12.7	13.3
Fencing														
Moderately		3.3	3.6	4.0	4.3	4.6	5.0	5.3	5.7	6.0	6.3	6.7	7.0	7.3
Vigorously		6.6	7.3	8.0	8.7	9.4	10.0	10.7	11.4	12.1	12.7	13.4	14.1	14.8

APPENDIX B *(continued)*

APPROXIMATE CALORIC EXPENDITURE PER MINUTE FOR VARIOUS PHYSICAL ACTIVITIES

BODY WEIGHT IN KILOGRAMS	45	50	55	59	64	68	73	77	82	86	91	95	100
BODY WEIGHT IN POUNDS	100	110	120	130	140	150	160	170	180	190	200	210	220
Football													
Moderate	3.3	3.6	4.0	4.3	4.6	5.0	5.3	5.7	6.0	6.3	6.7	7.0	7.3
Touch, vigorous	5.5	6.1	6.6	7.2	7.8	8.3	8.9	9.4	10.0	10.6	11.1	11.7	12.2
Golf													
Twosome (carry clubs)	3.6	4.0	4.4	4.7	5.1	5.4	5.8	6.2	6.6	6.9	7.3	7.6	8.0
Foursome (carry clubs)	2.7	3.0	3.3	3.5	3.8	4.1	4.4	4.6	4.9	5.2	5.4	5.7	6.0
Power-cart	1.9	2.1	2.3	2.5	2.7	2.9	3.1	3.3	3.5	3.7	3.9	4.1	4.3
Handball													
Moderate	6.5	7.2	7.8	8.5	9.2	9.9	10.5	11.2	11.9	12.5	13.2	13.8	14.5
Competitive	7.7	8.4	9.2	10.0	10.8	11.5	12.3	13.1	13.9	14.7	15.4	16.2	17.0
Hiking, pack (3 mph)	4.5	5.0	5.4	5.9	6.3	6.8	7.3	7.7	8.2	8.6	9.1	9.5	10.0
Hockey, field	5.0	6.7	7.3	7.9	8.5	9.1	9.7	10.3	10.9	11.5	12.1	12.7	13.3
Hockey, ice	6.6	7.3	8.0	8.7	9.4	10.0	10.7	11.4	12.1	12.7	13.4	14.1	14.8
Horseback riding													
Walk	1.9	2.1	2.3	2.5	2.7	2.9	3.1	3.3	3.5	3.7	3.9	4.1	4.3
Sitting to trot	2.7	3.0	3.3	3.5	3.8	4.1	4.4	4.6	4.9	5.2	5.4	5.7	6.0
Posting to trot	4.2	4.6	5.1	5.5	5.9	6.4	6.8	7.2	7.6	8.1	8.5	8.9	9.4
Gallop	5.7	6.3	6.9	7.5	8.1	8.7	9.3	9.8	10.4	11.0	11.6	12.2	12.8

APPENDIX B *(continued)*

APPROXIMATE CALORIC EXPENDITURE PER MINUTE FOR VARIOUS PHYSICAL ACTIVITIES

BODY WEIGHT IN KILOGRAMS	45	50	55	59	64	68	73	77	82	86	91	95	100
BODY WEIGHT IN POUNDS	100	110	120	130	140	150	160	170	180	190	200	210	220
Jogging (see Running)													
Judo	8.5	9.3	10.2	11.0	11.9	12.8	13.6	14.5	15.4	16.2	17.1	17.9	18.8
Karate	8.5	9.3	10.2	11.0	11.9	12.8	13.6	14.5	15.4	16.2	17.1	17.9	18.8
Mountain climbing	6.5	7.2	7.8	8.5	9.2	9.8	10.5	11.2	11.8	12.5	13.1	13.8	14.5
Paddle ball	5.7	6.3	6.9	7.5	8.1	8.7	9.3	9.8	10.4	11.0	11.6	12.2	12.8
Racquetball	6.5	7.1	7.8	8.4	9.1	9.8	10.4	11.1	11.7	12.4	13.0	13.7	14.4
Roller skating (9 mph)	4.2	4.6	5.1	5.5	5.9	6.4	6.8	7.2	7.6	8.1	8.5	8.9	9.4
Running (steady state)													
(mph) (min/mile)													
5.0 12:00	6.0	6.6	7.3	7.9	8.5	9.1	9.7	10.3	10.9	11.6	12.2	12.8	13.4
5.5 10:55	6.7	7.3	8.0	8.7	9.4	10.0	10.7	11.4	12.1	12.8	13.4	14.1	14.8
6.0 10:00	7.2	8.0	8.7	9.5	10.2	10.9	11.7	12.4	13.1	13.8	14.6	15.4	16.1
7.0 8:35	8.5	9.3	10.2	11.0	11.9	12.8	13.6	14.5	15.4	16.2	17.1	17.9	18.8
8.0 7:30	9.7	10.7	11.6	12.6	13.6	14.6	15.6	16.6	17.6	18.5	19.5	20.5	21.5
9.0 6:40	10.8	11.9	12.9	14.0	15.1	16.2	17.3	18.4	19.5	20.6	21.7	22.8	23.9
10.0 6:00	12.1	13.3	14.5	15.7	17.0	18.2	19.4	20.7	21.9	23.1	24.2	25.4	26.7
11.0 5:28	13.3	14.6	16.0	17.3	18.7	20.0	21.4	22.7	24.1	25.4	26.8	28.1	29.5
12.0 5:00	14.5	16.0	17.4	18.9	20.4	21.9	23.3	24.8	26.3	27.8	29.2	30.7	32.2

Appendix B *(continued)*

Approximate Caloric Expenditure Per Minute For Various Physical Activities

Body Weight in Kilograms	45	50	55	59	64	68	73	77	82	86	91	95	100
Body Weight in Pounds	100	110	120	130	140	150	160	170	180	190	200	210	220
Skating, ice (9 mph)	4.2	4.6	5.1	5.5	5.9	6.4	6.8	7.2	7.6	8.1	8.5	8.9	9.4
Skiing, cross-country													
(mph) (min/mile)													
2.5 24:00	5.0	5.5	6.0	6.5	7.0	7.5	8.0	8.5	9.0	9.5	10.0	10.6	11.1
4.0 15:00	6.5	7.2	7.8	8.5	9.2	9.9	10.5	11.2	11.9	12.5	13.2	13.8	14.5
5.0 12:00	7.7	8.4	9.2	10.0	10.8	11.5	12.3	13.1	13.9	14.7	15.4	16.2	17.0
Skiing, downhill	6.5	7.2	7.8	8.5	9.2	9.9	10.5	11.2	11.9	12.5	13.2	13.8	14.5
Soccer	5.9	6.6	7.2	7.8	8.4	9.0	9.6	10.2	10.8	11.4	12.0	12.6	13.2
Squash													
Normal	6.7	7.3	8.0	8.7	9.5	10.1	10.8	11.5	12.2	12.9	13.5	14.2	14.9
Competition	7.7	8.4	9.2	10.0	10.8	11.5	12.3	13.1	13.9	14.7	15.4	16.2	17.0
Swimming (yards/mi)													
Backstroke													
25	2.5	2.8	3.0	3.3	3.5	3.8	4.0	4.3	4.5	4.8	5.1	5.3	5.6
30	3.5	3.9	4.2	4.6	4.9	5.3	5.6	6.0	6.4	6.7	7.1	7.4	7.8
35	4.5	5.0	5.4	5.9	6.3	6.8	7.3	7.7	8.2	8.6	9.1	9.5	10.0
40	5.5	6.1	6.6	7.2	7.8	8.3	8.9	9.4	10.0	10.6	11.1	11.7	12.2

APPENDIX B *(continued)*

APPROXIMATE CALORIC EXPENDITURE PER MINUTE FOR VARIOUS PHYSICAL ACTIVITIES

BODY WEIGHT IN KILOGRAMS	45	50	55	59	64	68	73	77	82	86	91	95	100
BODY WEIGHT IN POUNDS	100	110	120	130	140	150	160	170	180	190	200	210	220
Swimming (yards/mi) *(continued)*													
Breaststroke													
20	3.1	3.5	3.8	4.1	4.5	4.8	5.1	5.4	5.7	6.0	6.4	6.7	7.0
30	4.7	5.2	5.7	6.2	6.7	7.1	7.6	8.1	8.6	9.1	9.5	10.0	10.5
40	6.3	7.0	7.6	8.3	8.9	9.6	10.2	10.9	11.5	12.2	12.8	13.5	14.1
Front crawl													
20	3.1	3.5	3.8	4.1	4.5	4.8	5.1	5.4	5.7	6.0	6.4	6.7	7.0
25	4.0	4.4	4.8	5.2	5.6	6.0	6.4	6.8	7.2	7.6	8.0	8.4	8.8
35	4.8	5.4	5.9	6.4	6.8	7.3	7.8	8.3	8.8	9.2	9.7	10.2	10.7
45	5.7	6.3	6.9	7.5	8.1	8.7	9.3	9.8	10.4	11.0	11.6	12.2	12.8
50	7.0	7.7	8.5	9.2	9.9	10.6	11.3	12.0	12.8	13.5	14.2	14.9	15.6
Table tennis	3.4	3.8	4.1	4.5	4.8	5.2	5.5	5.9	6.3	6.6	7.0	7.3	7.7
Tennis													
Singles (recreational)	5.0	5.5	6.0	6.5	7.0	7.5	8.0	8.5	9.0	9.5	10.0	10.6	11.1
Competition	6.4	7.1	7.7	8.4	9.1	9.8	10.4	11.1	11.8	12.4	13.1	13.7	14.4
Volleyball													
Moderate recreational	2.9	3.2	3.5	3.8	4.1	4.4	4.7	5.0	5.3	5.6	5.9	6.1	6.4
Vigorous, competition	6.5	7.1	7.8	8.4	9.1	9.8	10.4	11.1	11.7	12.4	13.0	13.7	14.4

APPENDIX B *(continued)*

APPROXIMATE CALORIC EXPENDITURE PER MINUTE FOR VARIOUS PHYSICAL ACTIVITIES

BODY WEIGHT IN KILOGRAMS		45	50	55	59	64	68	73	77	82	86	91	95	100
BODY WEIGHT IN POUNDS		100	110	120	130	140	150	160	170	180	190	200	210	220
Walking														
(mph)	(min/mile)													
2.0	30:00	2.1	2.3	2.5	2.8	3.0	3.2	3.4	3.6	3.9	4.1	4.3	4.5	4.7
3.0	20:00	2.7	3.0	3.3	3.5	3.8	4.1	4.4	4.6	4.9	5.2	5.4	5.7	6.0
3.5	17:10	3.3	3.7	4.0	4.4	4.7	5.1	5.4	5.8	6.2	6.5	6.9	7.2	7.6
4.0	15:00	4.2	4.6	5.1	5.5	5.9	6.4	6.8	7.2	7.6	8.1	8.5	8.9	9.4
4.5	13.20	4.7	5.2	5.7	6.2	6.7	7.1	7.6	8.1	8.6	9.1	9.5	10.0	10.5
5.0	12:00	5.4	6.0	6.5	7.1	7.7	8.2	8.7	9.2	9.8	10.4	10.9	11.5	12.0
5.4	11:10	6.2	6.9	7.5	8.2	8.8	9.5	10.1	10.3	11.4	12.1	12.7	13.4	14.0
5.8	10:20	7.7	8.4	9.2	10.0	10.8	11.5	12.3	13.1	13.9	14.7	15.4	16.2	17.0
Water skiing		5.0	5.5	6.0	6.5	7.0	7.5	8.0	8.5	9.0	9.5	10.0	10.6	11.1
Weight training		5.2	5.7	6.2	6.8	7.3	7.8	8.3	8.9	9.4	9.9	10.5	11.0	11.5
Wrestling		8.5	9.3	10.2	11.0	11.9	12.8	13.6	14.5	15.4	16.2	17.1	17.9	18.8

Note: The energy cost, in calories, will vary for different physical activities for a given individual depending on several factors. For example, the caloric cost of bicycling will vary depending on the type of bicycle, going uphill or downhill, and wind resistance. Walking with hand weights or ankle weights will increase energy output. Thus, the values expressed here are approximations and may be increased or decreased depending upon factors that influence energy cost.

Index

D

E

F

G

H

W

Z